WOMEN ON THE VERGE

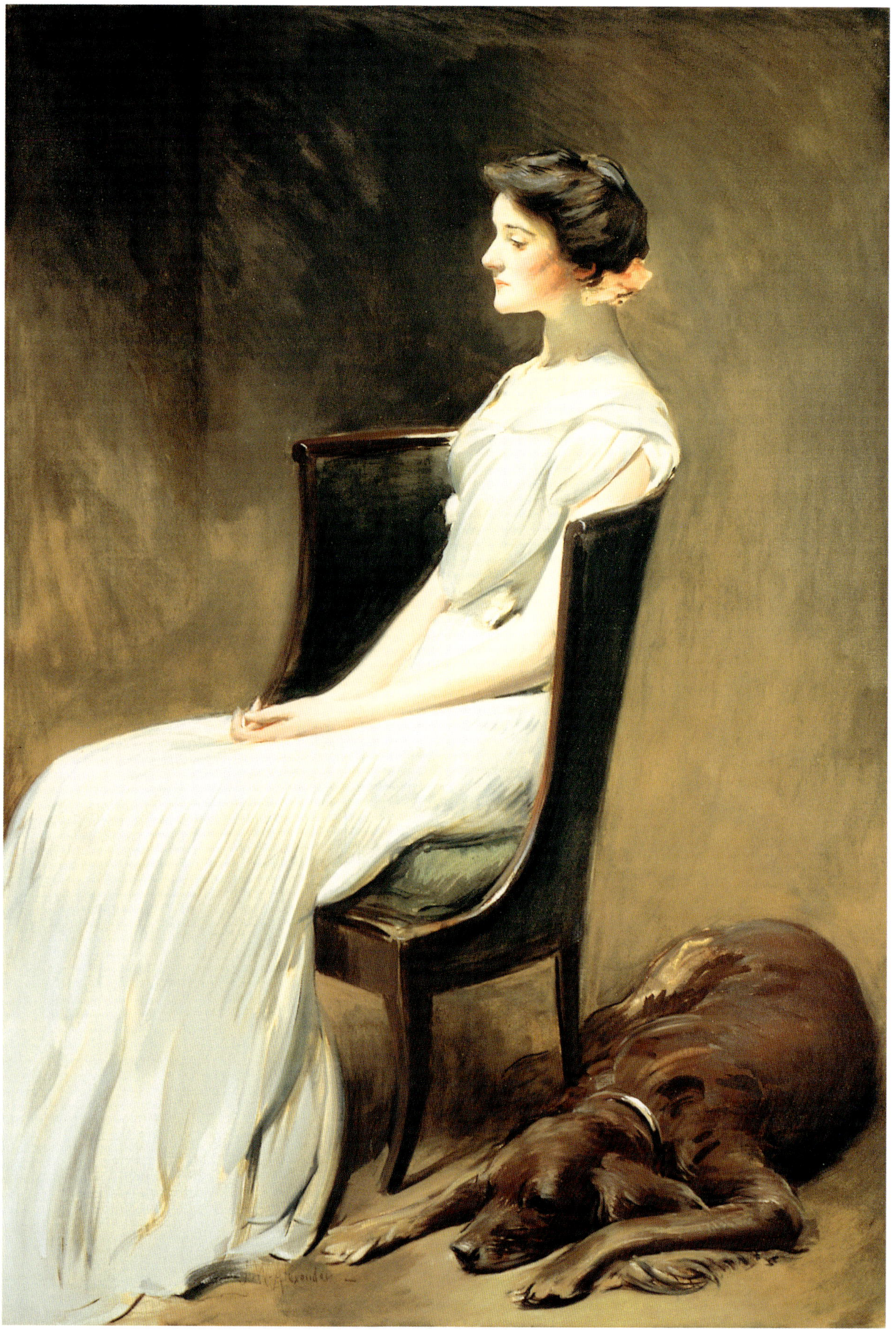

WOMEN *on the* VERGE

THE CULTURE OF NEURASTHENIA
IN NINETEENTH-CENTURY AMERICA

Essays by KATHERINE WILLIAMS,
ZACHARY ROSS, KATHLEEN SPIES,
AMANDA GLESMANN, *and* CLAIRE PERRY

With an introduction by
WANDA M. CORN

THE IRIS & B. GERALD CANTOR CENTER FOR VISUAL ARTS AT STANFORD UNIVERSITY

This book accompanies the exhibition *Women on the Verge:
The Culture of Neurasthenia in Nineteenth-Century America*
held at the Iris & B. Gerald Cantor Center for Visual Arts
at Stanford University November 11, 2004–February 6, 2005.
The exhibition, the catalogue, and related programs
are made possible by the Mariposa Fund and the
Halperin Exhibitions Fund.

FRONT COVER: Thomas Wilmer Dewing,
Lady in White (No. 2.), c. 1910. Oil on canvas,
22⅜ × 21⅜ in. Smithsonian American
Art Museum. Gift of John Gellatly.

FRONTISPIECE: John White Alexander, *Portrait
of Miss Dorothy Roosevelt (Mrs. Langdon Geer)*,
1901–1902. Oil on canvas, 60 × 40 in.
Schwarz Gallery, Philadelphia.

LIBRARY OF CONGRESS CATALOGUING-IN-PUBLICATION DATA

Ross, Zachary.

Women on the verge: the culture of neurasthenia in
nineteenth-century America / essays by Katherine Williams,
Zachary Ross, Kathleen Spies, Amanda Glesmann, Claire
Perry; with an introduction by Wanda M. Corn.

    p. cm.

Includes bibliographical references.

ISBN 0-937031-25-9 (pbk. : alk. paper)

1. Art and mental illness—Exhibitions.   2. Neurasthenia
in art—Exhibitions.   3. Women in art—Exhibitions.
4. Painting, American—19th century—Exhibitions.
5. Women—Mental health—United States—History—
19th century—Exhibitions.   6. Neurasthenia—United
States—History—19th century—Exhibitions.   I. Williams,
Katherine.   II. Glesmann, Amanda.   III. Spies, Kathleen.
IV. Perry, Claire.   V. Title.

    N71.5.R67 2004

    700'.45274'0973—dc22

                            2004042173

CONTENTS

FOREWORD

The development of the exhibition and catalogue *Women on the Verge: The Culture of Neurasthenia in Nineteenth-Century America* generated spirited conversations among the Cantor Arts Center curators and our project team. Much of the discussion focused on the distinct similarities between the "culture of neurasthenia" that existed a century ago and trends of late twentieth- and early twenty-first-century America, referred to by some as "the Prozac nation." Writers, social critics, educators, and the medical establishment of both eras believed the stress of modern life has a damaging effect on mental and physical health. In the late nineteenth century, women were considered to be more vulnerable than men to states of mental and physical exhaustion induced by crowded cities, industrial noise, and pressing time schedules. Women were also thought to be physically more fragile than men and particularly susceptible to the disease of neurasthenia.

Eight important paintings, generously loaned by the Smithsonian American Art Museum in Washington, D.C., and complemented by related materials, form the core of the *Women on the Verge* exhibition. These works portray well-to-do women of the late nineteenth century in a manner that came to be emblematic of the Gilded Age. Slender, meditative, and in a state of repose, the women in the paintings represent the refinement of their class. At the same time, their melancholy expressions and lassitude connect them to contemporary descriptions of neurasthenia, an illness that many nineteenth-century physicians believed had reached epidemic proportions in the United States.

The paintings and other visual material in *Women on the Verge* embody nineteenth-century debates over the character of women and their changing political, social, and economic roles. This debate is as timely today as it was at the end of the nineteenth century as we continue to confront the issues of women's reproductive rights, gender discrimination in many areas of employment, and the relative lack of attention given to women's health issues by the medical community.

It is my pleasure to thank the three women who collaborated to realize this project: Dr. Claire Perry, Curator of American Art at the Cantor Arts Center; Dr. Katherine Williams, a psychiatrist at the Women's Wellness Clinic at Stanford University Medical Center; and Amanda Glesmann, doctoral candidate in the Department of Art and Art History at Stanford. Elizabeth Broun, Director of the Smithsonian American Art Museum, helped to make the exhibition possible through the generous loan of the core paintings. Another colleague, Professor Wanda M. Corn from Stanford's Department of Art and Art History, has been a valuable guide at critical junctures and contributed the illuminating introduction to this collection of essays. Bernard Barryte, chief curator, expertly shepherded this rich catalogue through the press in collaboration with the production team at Wilsted & Taylor Publishing Services, and Jeanie Lawrence, Curatorial Assistant, did an outstanding job with all aspects of the loans, installation, and catalogue for the exhibition. The registrarial responsibilities for the exhibition were in Katie Clifford's capable hands, while Sarah Miller worked out the complexities of budget and scheduling. I also wish to thank the other lenders and individuals, including the Halperin Exhibitions Fund, that contributed to the success of this project, and to express our gratitude for the generosity of the Mariposa Fund for support of the catalogue.

Thomas K. Seligman
JOHN & JILL FREIDENRICH DIRECTOR

WOMEN ON THE VERGE

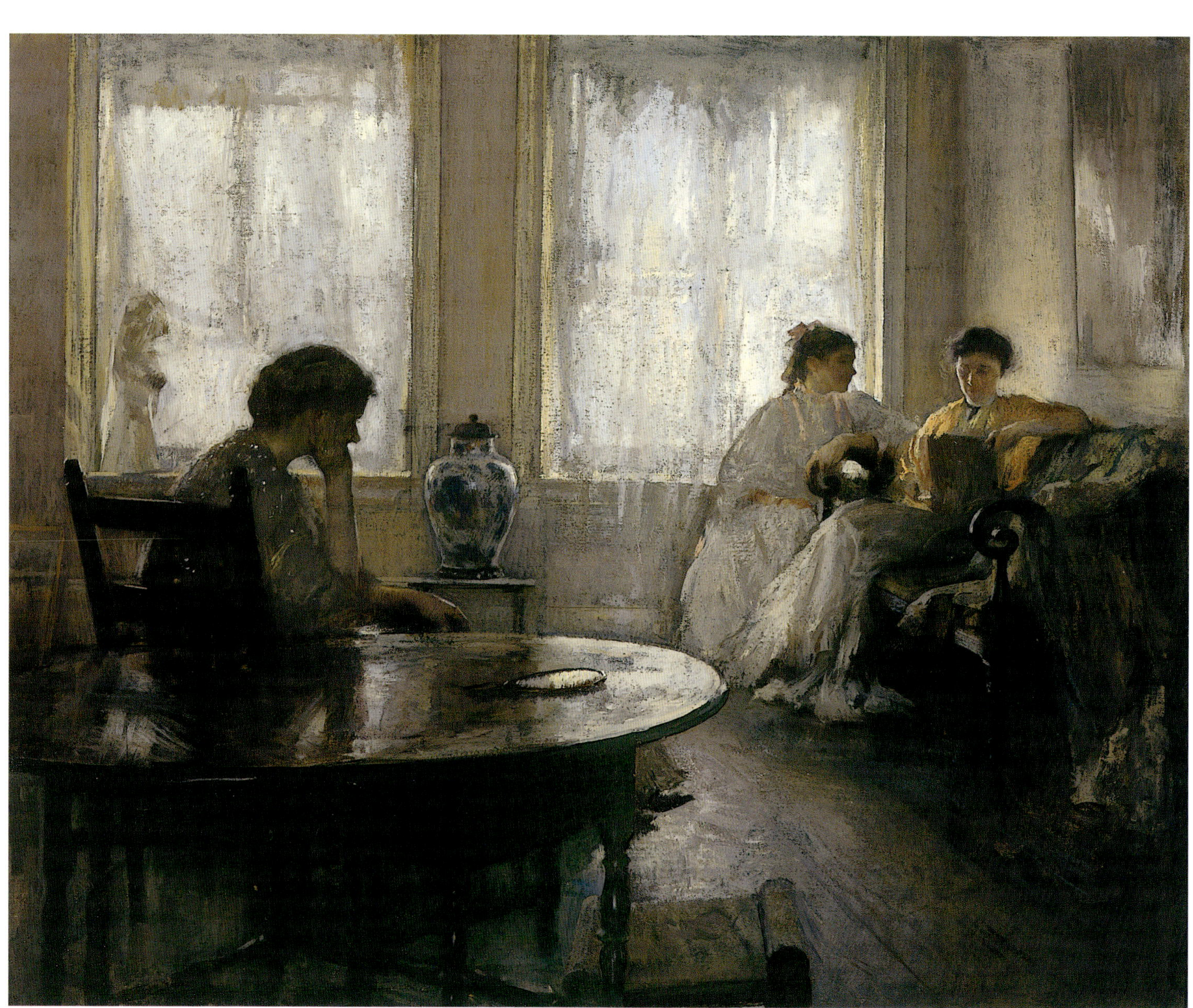

"BRAIN FAG"

Have you brain fag, no appetite, insomnia?
Are you irritable? Has your brain lost its alertness?
PROMOTIONAL BROCHURE, C. 1905
SAGAMORE BEACH INVESTMENT ASSOCIATION

In my family, we go to the beach house to relieve "brain fag." We came to know this late Victorian phrase through the opening lines of a real estate brochure luring New Englanders to a new beachside development in Sagamore Highlands, Massachusetts, some fifty miles southeast of Boston. The commercial project never materialized, but my family has summered on a few of the original lots for nearly sixty years. Sunny and quiet days at the seashore continue to be a splendid antidote to the stresses and strains of modern urban life that people once considered the cause of "brain fag."

This book and the exhibition it accompanies explore this malady in both medical science and period imagery. Brain fag—or "neurasthenia," to use the more common term—was no laughing matter a century ago. Doctors and patients alike believed that the harsh conditions of modern industrial society had generated new nervous disorders afflicting mature men and women. The symptoms varied but included an inability to sleep, a loss of appetite, listlessness, and a variety of aches and pains. The cures were equally diverse and often experimental. And they were deeply gendered. Men were encouraged to seek new climes and to be active out of doors, be it on the plains of the West or in the forests of the East. The usual prescription for women was literally the opposite, an enforced period in bed with little or no activity or interaction with others. Alternative therapies included extreme diets and electrical shocks.

In that middle- and upper-class women were thought to be especially susceptible to nervous diseases and that neurasthenic women endured what appear today to be harsh therapies, this all-inclusive medical condition has been a rich topic for recent scholars of women's history and for those looking anew at the complexities of American culture during the Gilded Age. As a "period disease," common from the 1870s into the early twentieth century, female neurasthenia seems related to, if not caused by, tumultuous changes reorienting women's lives. During these decades women increasingly lived in cities and ventured out of the private sphere of the home into a range of public spaces. Younger women attending colleges and universities could contemplate paid professions such as teaching, office work, writing, or artistic endeavors. Married women, especially those with means, were moving into club life, charitable organizations, and art associations.

FIG. 1 [*facing*] Edmund Charles Tarbell, *Girls Reading*, 1907. Oil on canvas, 25 × 30 in. Collection of Deborah Shein.

Because of the increasingly vocal suffrage movement, a national campaign that focused on woman's unequal status outside the home and the need for laws granting her the right to vote, women of all ages, races, and religious persuasions were thinking anew about their place in American society.

The ideology of female primacy in the home had sustained many women throughout the nineteenth century, particularly middle- and upper-class women, whose lives and behaviors were governed by deep-seated conventions. They had been raised to be wives, mothers, and ladies and lived by the laws of gentility that afforded limited opportunities to move outside the social circles to which they had been born. As women found themselves with new opportunities for higher education and public activities, their role as "ladies of the home" became a matter of national debate and anxiety. When women expressed desire for new freedoms, they often faced a backlash from both men and women seeking to maintain the home as the primary female sphere. Women were often bewildered, frightened, and depressed by the disconnect between unprecedented opportunities and the genteel restraints that kept them in their accustomed place. Psychological counseling was not yet common, and formal support groups to work through collective problems did not exist. Journals and the daily press included little self-help literature dedicated to helping women learn how to express and fulfill growing ambitions and desires.

Female neurasthenia, recent scholars have shown, was linked to these broader currents of disruption and realignment of gender roles. To demonstrate the historical connections between cultural repression and women's mental breakdowns, literary scholars have reprinted vintage literature authored by women about female nervous disorders. Today many have their first encounters with late nineteenth-century neurasthenic women when reading modern editions of Kate Chopin's novella *The Awakening* (1899) and Charlotte Perkins Gilman's short story *The Yellow Wallpaper*[1] (1892; fig. 2). Both are brilliant accounts of women driven to the depths of despair by conventional marriages and the unsympathetic social codes that keep the one from painting, the other from writing. In *The Awakening*,

Edna Pontellier finds the routines of her respectable family unbearable; when she asserts her independence and leaves her husband and children to be an artist, society condemns her. Eventually she is so mentally conflicted that, to find peace and equilibrium, she does what so many women do in nineteenth-century literature: she takes her own life.

In *The Yellow Wallpaper*, an autobiographical story, Charlotte Perkins Gilman describes the horrific psychological and sensory deprivations women endured when they underwent a "rest cure" for their "nervous disorders." Her husband-doctor prescribes a summer of bed rest in a third-floor nursery with barred windows. She is to have no visitors other than her husband and his sister, who tends to her housekeeping. To calm what her husband diagnoses as "temporary nervous depression—a slight hysterical tendency," Gilman is forbidden all activities including writing, her metier.[2] Solitary confinement slowly erodes her self-confidence and her sanity. All she has to look at and keep her company are the florid arabesques of the putrid yellow wallpaper in her room. As she sinks into madness, the patterns on the ugly wallpaper begin to convulse; soon she is hallucinating, seeing the body of a woman held captive behind the paper's patterns. Driven finally into a psychotic state by her "cure," she attacks the walls, clawing at the decaying wallpaper to free the imprisoned woman. Her room, its decaying wallpaper, and the bars on the windows become a complex metaphor for the lunacy of the rest cure and of the medical profession that prescribed it.

Artists of the era, particularly white males of the Northeast, contributed imagery that helped enforce the medical discourse of neurasthenia. Expert opinion had it that women, given their monthly cycles and child-bearing bodies, were much more at risk than men for brain diseases. Painters and art photographers rarely depicted ill women, but they created body types and a body language that conformed to the medical profession's belief that women were physiologically and psychologically weak. Thomas Dewing, for example,

FIG. 2 *The Yellow Wall-paper*, 1892. Reproduced from *The New England Magazine* (January 1892). Courtesy of Cornell University Library, Making of America Digital Collection.

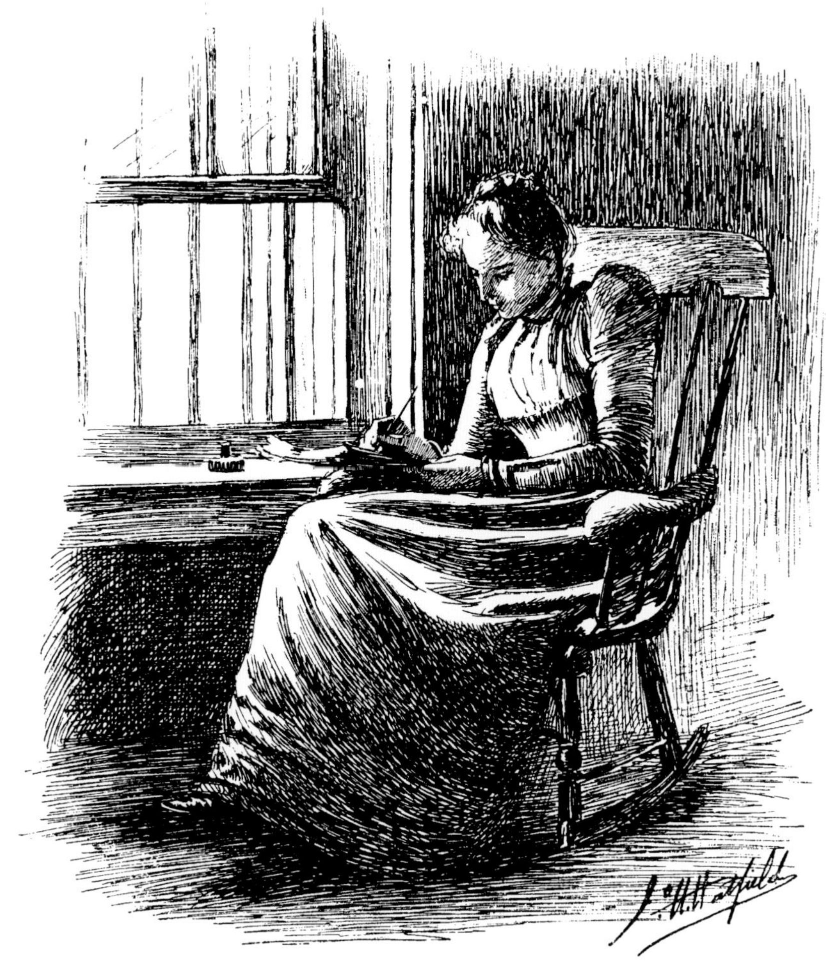

"I am sitting by the Window in this Atrocious Nursery."

THE YELLOW WALL-PAPER.

By Charlotte Perkins Stetson.

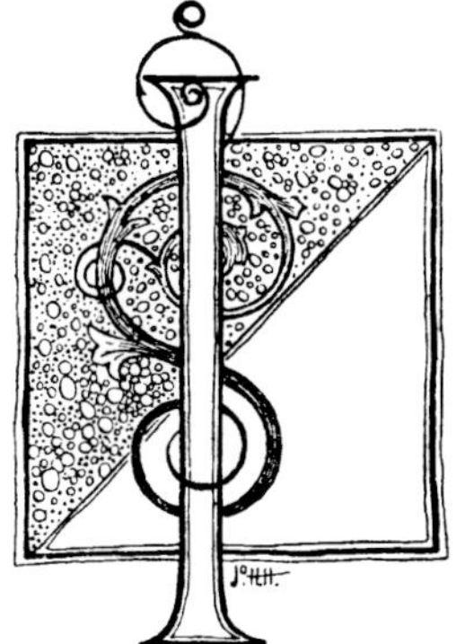

IT is very seldom that mere ordinary people like John and myself secure ancestral halls for the summer.

A colonial mansion, a hereditary estate, I would say a haunted house, and reach the height of romantic felicity — but that would be asking too much of fate !

Still I will proudly declare that there is something queer about it.

Else, why should it be let so cheaply? And why have stood so long untenanted?

John laughs at me, of course, but one expects that in marriage.

John is practical in the extreme. He has no patience with faith, an intense horror of superstition, and he scoffs openly at any talk of things not to be felt and seen and put down in figures.

John is a physician, and *perhaps* — (I would not say it to a living soul, of course, but this is dead paper and a great relief to my mind —) *perhaps* that is one reason I do not get well faster.

You see he does not believe I am sick ! And what can one do?

pictured women as exquisitely poetic creatures, with long languid bodies, resting impassively in empty interior settings. Other artists, such as Edmund Tarbell, Frank Benson, Joseph DeCamp, and William Paxton of the so-called Boston School, portrayed women as having acutely sensitive natures or doing small domestic chores in overarching interiors that engulf them, as if holding them under a spell (see fig. 1). They are beautiful beings often lost in private reverie and disengaged from any life taking place outside the walls of their home. These pictures reinforce the period literature about female neurasthenia in which women were encouraged to rest and avoid stress and "brain work."

Women on the Verge builds on recent art history that has isolated and identified the trope of withdrawn, genteel women in domestic interiors. It also contributes to the growing literature about female neurasthenia during the Gilded Age. The first essay, by Katherine Williams, a psychiatrist specializing in women's mental health, clearly maps neurasthenia as it was understood by neurologists and other medical authorities during the last half of the nineteenth century. She explains how physicians linked the disease to the physiological structure of the female body and prescribed a range of therapies: electric shocks, extended vacations, and, most popularly, the rest cure. Williams argues that medical expertise today sees the neurasthenia of yesterday as an obsolete diagnosis. What was once an all-inclusive nervous disorder now includes many different mental or physical conditions: affective disorders, including major depression and bipolar disorder; and anxiety disorders, including obsessive-compulsive disorder, eating disorders, thyroid diseases, or chronic fatigue syndrome. Just as with neurasthenia, these illnesses are more common in women than in men, but they are no longer attached, as they were a hundred years ago, to stereotypes that women are physiologically the weaker, more emotional, and more sensitive sex.

Essays by Zachary Ross and Kathleen Spies link the fine art of the period—particularly paintings of female figures in domestic interiors—to the culture of neurasthenia. Ross finds the widespread depiction of the stilled and quiet female at home to be intimately connected to the pervasive belief that brain fag was caused by excessive activity, intellectual work, and over-excitement. The antidote, recommended by not only doctors but also self-help literature, was to rest and completely disengage from urban distractions. The late nineteenth-century American paintings of quiet women, Ross argues, were consonant with both the diagnosis of and the cures for nervous disorders. In their repose and calm, women-at-home images modeled the behaviors doctors recommended to stave off nervous disfunctions. These poetically quiescent images also evoked in viewers an aesthetic reverie that was itself therapeutic. As Matisse would later say about his paintings, these images could be as soothing and comforting as an armchair after a hard day of work.

Spies looks specifically at the late portraiture of Thomas Eakins, in which female faces and bodies, as well as those of men, are weary, enervated, and prematurely aged. Eakins knew the disease well. Not only was he friendly with some of the Philadelphia doctors who specialized in this ailment, but he himself was diagnosed as a neurasthenic in 1886. On the recommendation of his doctor, he took a camping trip to the American West to alleviate his symptoms. Male professionals and intellectuals, Spies points out, were sometimes diagnosed as "cerebrasthenics," having "brain exhaustion" rather than the nervous exhaustion attributed to women. This called for an altogether different kind of cure, such as a change of scene and robust activities out of doors; men were encouraged to ingest fresh air and to be physically active.

Spies carefully points out the various signs of exhaustion that suffuse Eakins's portraits of both men and women and helps us decode the gendered ways these symptoms would have been read in their own time. When Eakins gave his female sitters drawn features, teary eyes, physical exhaustion, and an inward gaze, these characteristics could be taken as normal and natural in an age that viewed women as prone to nervous breakdown. But given that these portraits were painted by a male artist, they also suggested sexual submissiveness and partook in the "eroticized sick woman" image popular in the arts and literature of the time. When Eakins imbued his male sitters with the same vulnerabilities, Spies argues, the portraits registered differently. Viewers might have read withdrawn men as effeminate or homosexual, for instance, but also as endowed with intellectual intensity, profound sensitivity, and the disturbed genius and unrecognized heroism of the modern artist.

Amanda Glesmann's essay offers a vivid portrait of the Gibson Girl, whose appearance in the 1890s challenged a society that took it for granted that women were weak, men were strong, and modern life was dangerous to health and well-being. In Glesmann's study we sense the complexity of change in gender roles that festered at the *fin de siècle* a hundred years ago. The Gibson Girl, a newly imagined female prototype, offered a model of femininity that countered the passive and emotionally fragile women rendered by Dewing, Eakins, Tarbell, and others. Invented by Charles Dana Gibson, an illustrator for popular magazines, the Gibson Girl was young, independent, and physically active. She was an outdoor girl, bicycling, playing golf, swimming, ice-skating, and driving cars. Her strenuous activities, and her release from the domestic interior, meant that she, like the suffragists, upset the social order. Her sassy independence flew in the face of the dominant paradigm of middle- and upper-class women born and bred to gentility. As Glesmann explains, the Gibson Girl represented a model of youth but not of mature womanhood; she was a *girl*. Her emancipation from the confinement of the home was, the illustrations imply, a prenuptial privilege and a new avenue to marriage. The Gibson Girl took pride in her physical beauty, flirted shamelessly, and was generally, just like older generations, on the lookout for a marriageable beau. In her desire to marry, she demonstrated her ties to more traditional feminine ideals and offered some comfort to men and women worried that her alternative ways of growing up might shatter the traditions of home and the family.

Even with such reassurances, however, the creation and popularity of the Gibson Girl evidenced the expansion of roles women began to imagine in the late nineteenth century. On the one hand, this reordering of female potential could bring on depression and other neurasthenic illnesses. On the other hand, the healthy and active Gibson Girl suggested flaws in the medical and cultural construction of women's bodies as consti-

tutionally weak and inherently susceptible to nervous disorders.

In the catalogue's final essay, Claire Perry details some of the rich social history of women's (as opposed to girls') activities that, along with the Gibson Girl's vigor and dynamism, helped erode the rigid codes by which many nineteenth-century women lived their lives. The historical records of upper-class women in the Gilded Age, Perry reminds us, show them to be far more active participants in the public sphere than paintings of women in the home suggest. Many woman volunteers worked hard to better the conditions for their sex. Suffragists worked for legislation granting women the right to vote; woman activists argued for shortened workdays for female laborers and for the abolition of child labor; and club members raised money for a wide variety of charitable and benevolent causes. Women helped establish women's colleges and forced open the doors of male schools to female students. These kinds of social activities and leadership roles, along with the new freedoms granted the American girl, were recorded in newspapers, documentary photographs, and letters but rarely inspired the work of fine artists. Eventually, if slowly, these forays of mature women into public life effected changes in gender roles. Post–Gibson Girl generations would have advantages and options their mothers never did. Rest cures would become extinct, and neurasthenia, as it was understood in the late nineteenth century, a discredited disease.

Wanda M. Corn
STANFORD UNIVERSITY

Notes

1. Kate Chopin, *The Awakening*, 1899, was republished in 1932 but did not attract a large readership until 1969 when it appeared in Per Seyersted's *The Complete Works of Kate Chopin* (Louisiana State University). See *Kate Chopin: The Awakening and Selected Stories*, ed. Sandra M. Gilbert (New York: Penguin Books, 1984), 43–176. Charlotte Perkins Gilman, *The Yellow Wallpaper*, 1892, was printed in 1899, in 1920, and then in another edition edited by Elaine R. Hedges (Old Westbury, NY: The Feminist Press, 1973). The first edition was published with "wallpaper" spelled differently than in later editions and with the pseudonym Charlotte Perkins Stetson.

2. Hedges, ed., *Yellow Wallpaper*, 10.

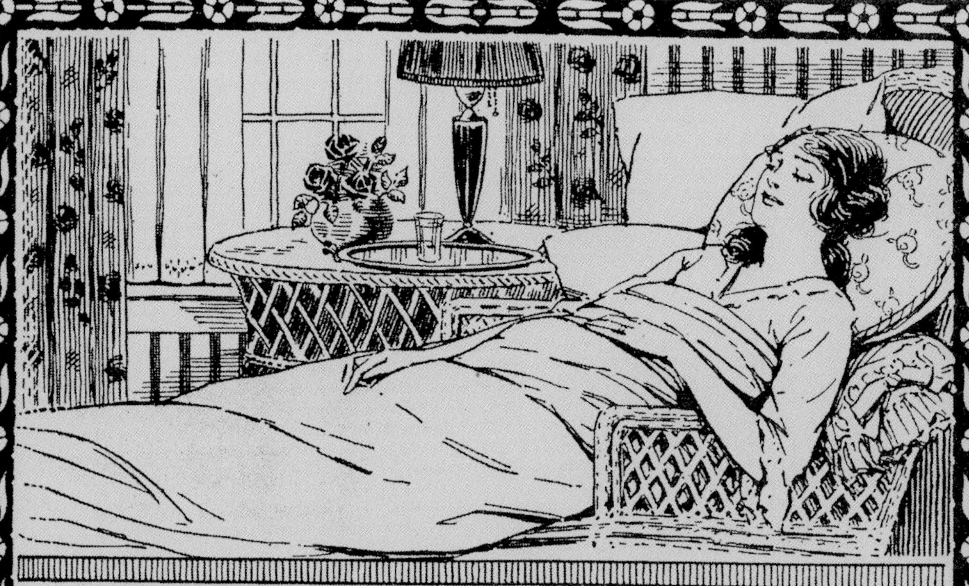

Nervous Breakdown

"I am so nervous it seems as though I should fly"—"My nerves are all on edge"—"I wish I were dead." How often have we heard these expressions or others quite as extravagant from some loved one who has been brought to this state by some female trouble which has slowly developed until the nerves can no longer stand up under it. No woman should allow herself to drift into this condition without giving that good old-fashioned root and herb remedy Lydia E. Pinkham's Vegetable Compound a trial.

Read the Letters of These Two Women.

North East, Md.—"I was in ill health four or five years and doctored with one doctor after another but none helped me. I was irregular and had such terrible pain in my back, lower part of my body and down each side that I had to go to bed three or four days every month. I was very nervous, tired, could not sleep and could not eat without getting sick. A friend asked me to take Lydia E. Pinkham's Vegetable Compound and I am sorry I did not take it sooner for it has helped me wonderfully. I don't have to go to bed with the pain, can eat without being sick and have more strength. I recommend your medicine and you are at liberty to publish my testimonial."—ELIZABETH WEAVER, R. R. 2, North East, Md.

Minneapolis, Minn.—"I was run down and nervous, could not rest at night and was more tired in the morning than when I went to bed. I have two children, the youngest three months old and it was drudgery to care for them as I felt so irritable and generally worn out. From lack of rest and appetite my baby did not get enough nourishment from my milk so I started to give him two bottle feedings a day. After taking three bottles of Lydia E. Pinkham's Vegetable Compound I felt like a new woman, full of life and energy. It is a pleasure to care for my children, and I am very happy with them and feel fine. I nurse my baby exclusively again, and can't say too much for your medicine."—MRS. A. L. MILLER, 2633 E. 24th St., Minneapolis, Minn.

Nervous, Ailing Women Should Rely Upon

Lydia E. Pinkham's Vegetable Compound

KATHERINE WILLIAMS

AMERICAN WOMEN AND "NERVOUSNESS"
NEURASTHENIA THEN AND NOW

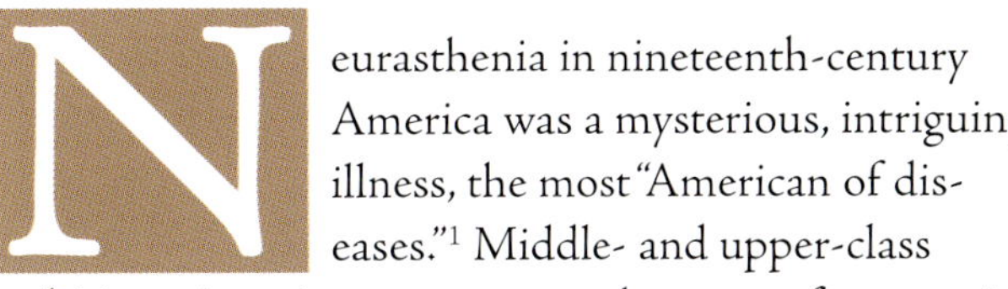

Neurasthenia in nineteenth-century America was a mysterious, intriguing illness, the most "American of diseases."[1] Middle- and upper-class ambitious American women, on the verge of new social, political, and educational spheres, were believed to be especially susceptible to this "nervous exhaustion"[2] (fig. 3). Through a modern psychiatric lens, neurasthenia can be seen as a drama between patients and doctors played out on the verge of a new century. While this drama is vividly evoked in the lasting artistic and literary expressions of the Gilded Age, many important details of the script are found in the actual medical texts and case records of neurasthenia. Close examination of the medical history of neurasthenia in women reveals an underlying story—the tension-filled connection between the mind and the body. This complex interface remains alive and challenging today in the modern specialties of psychiatry and gynecology. What factors brought neurasthenia to the medical and social forefront during this time and led it to be construed as so common and even fashionable? How was it diagnosed and treated in women? What insights can modern medicine provide into the true etiology of nineteenth-century neurasthenia, and how do recent advances in women's mental health research further illuminate this mysterious malady? Such questions guide our exploration into the medical history of neurasthenia and its role for "women on the verge."

Neurasthenia: Causes and Symptoms

Neurasthenia made its debut in 1869 when George Beard, MD, a well-respected neurologist, presented his original communication to the *Boston Medical and Surgical Journal*. In "Neurasthenia, or Nervous Exhaustion," he introduced the belief that nervous disorders were becoming more common because of the stress on the brain from urbanization and industrialization in post–Civil War America.[3] Beard's extensive and diverse list of symptoms included "general malaise, debility of all the functions, poor appetite, abiding weakness in the back and spine, fugitive neuralgic pains, hysteria, insomnia, hypochondriasis, disinclination for consecutive mental labor, severe and weakening attacks of sick headache and other analogous symptoms."[4] Over time, Beard became more specific in his classification system

FIG. 3 [*facing*] "Nervous Breakdown." Courtesy of Schlesinger Library.

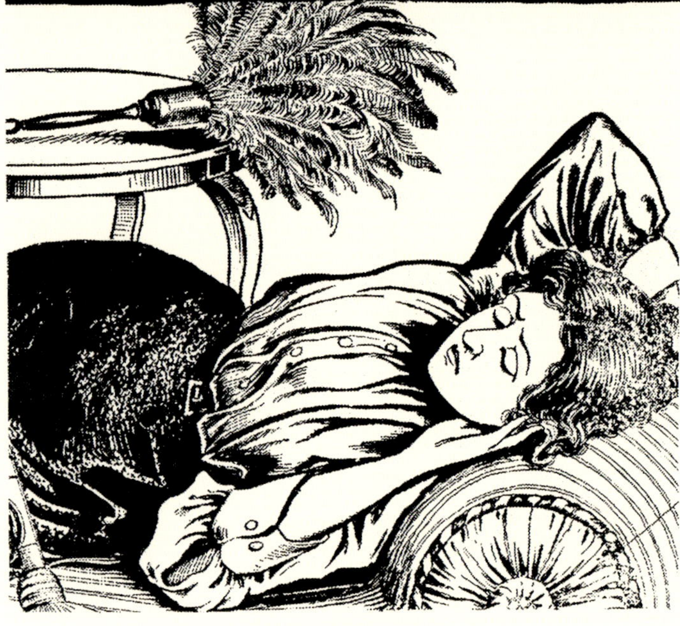

FIG. 4 "I'm Simply all Worn Out."
Courtesy of Schlesinger Library.

for neurasthenia, dividing it into six distinct categories: cerebrasthenia (exhaustion of the brain), myalasthenia (exhaustion of the spinal cord), digestive neurasthenia (nervous dyspepsia), sexual neurasthenia, traumatic neurasthenia, and hysterical neurasthenia.[5]

In 1881, in his popular book *American Nervousness: Its Causes and Consequences*, Beard wrote that neurasthenia had become so widespread in America, especially in the northern cities, "that there is no need of statistics."[6] He emphasized the popular medical view that women, especially middle- and upper-class women, were especially vulnerable to the ailment. "In civilized lands, women are more nervous, immeasurably than men,"[7] Beard wrote, and he asserted that lower-class women and Native American women ("the squaw") escaped the illness because of their lack of cultivation and refinement.[8] His descriptions of the typical female neurasthenic phenotype—"fine soft hair, delicate skin,

nicely chiseled features, long tapering extremities"— spoke to the status and fashionable nature of the illness[9] (fig. 4).

Beard and other medical authorities believed that the female reproductive system was intimately involved in the cause and effect of the increased prevalence of neurasthenia in women. The primacy of the female sexual organs in the minds of many medical writers of the time is reflected in the often-quoted 1870s physician's statement that it was "as if the Almighty in creating the female sex, had taken the uterus and built up a woman around it."[10] Uterine problems became a leading etiology of nineteenth-century neurasthenia, also called genito-urinary neurasthenia. While in the male, sexual neurasthenia was most frequently caused by "sexual excesses," including masturbation, in the female it was more often caused by pelvic pathology. "This is an exceedingly common form of neurasthenia," wrote a leading neurologist, James Jewell, in 1880. "In the female it arises chiefly from irritative diseases of the uterus and ovaries and sensitive parts within the pelvis."[11] Causes of pelvic pathology included infections such as gonorrhea, cervical and uterine malignancies, fibroids, and birth trauma.

The birthing process in America at the time of neurasthenia's debut was itself in the midst of major transformations. While in colonial America childbirth had primarily been part of the "women's sphere," childbirth for upper-class women at the cusp of the twentieth century had moved into a medical male sphere.[12] During the nineteenth century, obstetricians, mainly male, began to supplant the traditional midwife in home deliveries. Over time, middle- and upper-class women began to deliver their babies in hospital rooms, enticed by the promise of anesthesia and quicker deliveries, mainly through the use of forceps.[13] However, women were caught between this push for the medicalization of childbirth and the pull for natural childbirth, advocated by the health reform movement, which was made up increasingly of women.[14]

Thus, age-old anxieties surrounding childbirth took on new dimensions for middle- and upper-class nineteenth-century American women. As they battled their terror of labor pain and death, they also had to consider where and how to deliver their child, and whether the birth would be associated with protracted physical or mental morbidity, which included the specter of neurasthenia.[15] Beard stated, "How many, also, to whom the simple act of giving birth to a child opens the door to unnumbered woes; beginning with lacerations and relaxations, extending to displacements and ovarian imprisonments, and ending by setting the whole system on fire with neuralgias, tremors, etc and compelling a life-long slavery to sleeplessness, hysteria or insanity."[16]

Reproductive events, such as puberty, pregnancy, and menopause, even if uncomplicated by illness or trauma, were also considered important in the onset of neurasthenia because these bodily changes required so much energy. Since the nervous system was conceptualized as a "bank" and people were endowed with only a fixed amount of nerve force, or "nervous reserve," these reproductive cycle–related events were seen as a grave threat to women's mental health. As late as 1900, George Englemann, president of the American Gynecological Association, warned of the dangerous interface between psychiatry and gynecology:

> Many a young life is battered and forever crippled on the breakers of puberty; if it crosses these unharmed and is not dashed to pieces on the rock of childbirth, it may still ground on the ever-recurring shallows of menstruation, and lastly upon the final bar of the menopause ere protection is found in the unruffled waters of the harbor beyond the reach of sexual storms.[17]

Pregnancy, in particular, was thought to strain a woman's nervous system. "The process of parturition is everywhere the measure of nerve strength," declared Beard. "Had we no other barometer than this, we should know that civilization was paid for by nervousness, and that our cities are builded [sic] out of the life-force of their populations."[18] In the Victorian mindset, the pregnant mother had exceptional influence over her fetus. It was believed that a mother should stay calm and not upset her unborn child, and this advice could be found in medical texts and advice manuals.[19]

Because these reproductive events were so taxing to the naturally weaker female brain, physicians warned that too much "mental work" would further deplete a woman's reserves and derange the system even further.[20]

Even Margaret Cleaves, a rarity as a female physician, subscribed to this notion. In her paper "Neurasthenia and Its Relation to Diseases of Women" she observed, "In no country or time has there been so much would-be mental activity among women as here and now." This "craze for universal higher education of women," as well as increased social obligations, led to "drains upon their [women's] nervous systems."[21]

Physicians became especially concerned about the effects of "mental activity" on pubertal development and about the risk of decreased fertility. Medical experts asserted that the increased demands of secondary school education and the "craze for higher education" were responsible for delayed puberty, amenorrhea, and infertility. As recently as 1901, the physician William Darnall, in the *American Gynecological and Obstetrical Journal*, described these "highly cultured and accomplished" young women in the following way:

> The poor sufferer only adds another to the great army of neurasthenia and sexual incompetents, which furnish neurologists and gynecologists with so much of their material.... bright eyes have been dulled by the brain-fag [sic] and sweet temper transformed into irritability, crossness and hysteria, while the womanhood of the land is deteriorating physically.[22]

When medical writers worried about the decline in the "womanhood of the land," they were especially concerned about the decline in birthrates of white middle- and upper-class women. Major changes had occurred in family planning and birth control for these relatively well-off women, and by 1900 white women had an average of 3.56 children, compared to seven at the beginning of the eighteenth century. This decline is probably due to active family planning, including birth control and abortions, rather than to an epidemic of infertility.[23] Immigrant women, in contrast, continued to have large families, but their continued fecundity does not appear to have eased the minds of society physicians.

Consequently, a medical opinion emerged that placed the blame squarely on the rise of women in academics. In 1873, Edward H. Clarke, professor at Harvard University, published *Sex in Education, or, a Fair Chance for the Girls*, a treatise advocating that women should rest during their menstrual periods and avoid higher education.[24] Despite the fact that this was a time when women were making unprecedented advances in academic, business, and social reform, and studies were conducted that showed that these activities did not harm women's health,[25] Clarke's book was nevertheless quite popular. *Sex in Education* sold seventeen editions within the next thirteen years, and physicians continued to warn of the dangers of "mental work" in women despite the vociferous protestations of Clarke's many critics.[26]

Treatment of Neurasthenia

Neurasthenic therapy for women was based upon these converging theories of etiology and represents a carefully orchestrated treatment intervention that included attention to physiological, psychological, and social factors. Physiologically, treating physicians focused upon the local reproductive system, and middle- and upper-class women experienced the profession of gynecology itself "on the verge," with new developments in medicines, gynecological devices, and surgery. Treatment of a female neurasthenic often began with a manual examination, for as Beard stated, "No treatment of these cases is regarded in any sense as scientific where such examination is not made and where the proper local treatment is not employed."[27] Indeed, the Victorian gynecologic exam was itself a drama between doctor and patient, a subtext in the history of neurasthenia. While these exams were considered vitally important, they were hindered by concepts of propriety. Medical texts show physicians examining fully clothed women, and medical students were warned of the potential for sexual arousal induced by the speculum.[28]

Pathology on manual examination was a frequent finding; one physician complained, "The widespread mutilation … is so common, indeed, that we scarcely find a normal perineum after childbirth."[29] A displaced uterus, or prolapsed uterus due to birth trauma, was a recognized local cause of the symptoms of neurasthenia and mandated pessary placement. (Pessaries were intervaginal supporters, and women were availed of over one hundred types of pessary.)[30] Since corsets were

considered another cause of uterine displacement, women were also caught up in the drama of social reform.[31] Health and social welfare reformers, ranging from male and female physicians to the Women's Christian Temperance Union, called for women to stop wearing corsets, a major risk to female health.[32] Frances Willard, the president of the Women's Christian Temperance Movement, declared in 1892, "Niggardly waists and niggardly brains go together."[33]

By the last decades of the nineteenth century, scientists had learned that menstruation was dependent upon the presence of the ovaries, and, over time, the ovaries became recognized as a potential independent source of neurasthenia.[34] The weeks before menstruation were believed to be a high-risk time for either the onset or the exacerbation of neurasthenic complaints. After the first oophorectomy in 1809 for diseased organs, oophorectomies increased in frequency during the later half of the twentieth century and were used for the treatment of diseased minds as well.[35]

Patent medicines were another form of widely used "biological" treatments. Lydia Pinkham's Vegetable Compound was one of the most popular, and while it was originally sold for soothing female pelvic complaints, it became firmly identified with the larger scope of the "American disease," neurasthenia. Advertisements such as "Don't Blame Her" (fig. 5) reflected the prevailing medical opinion that women were predisposed to mental illness because of their sexual physiology. These ads reveal the popularization of medical theories: "It gives the womb and uterus the necessary strength to throw off the diseases which burden it, the nagging nerves are quieted, the sufferer becomes a rational being again, and can re-enter society with no fear of making a sad exhibition of herself."[36] Early Pinkham campaigns depicted middle- and upper-class women in fashionable attire unable to continue their social duties, thus promoting the image of neurasthenia as a disease of female refinement (fig. 6). Over time, other threats to female health, like higher education, were incorporated into the advertisements as well (fig. 7).

While Pinkham's patent medicines were targeted generally to wealthy, fashionable sufferers, the women who frequented the consulting rooms of elite physicians such as Beard were offered prescription medications as well. Prescription pharmacological approaches to neurasthenia included the liberal use of sedatives, such as chloral hydrate, as well as "general sedatives" like lithium bromide. "General tonics" were used to restore vitality and nerve force and included iron, phosphoric acid, coca, and zinc. Many of the tonics from the time contained generous doses of cod liver oil, which was believed to be especially useful for improving the functioning of the nervous system.[37]

Beard popularized electricity as yet another physiological treatment of neurasthenia. Three types of electrical current were used, depending upon the patient's symptoms: galvanic, faradic, and static. Galvanic appears to have been the strongest current and the one most frequently used, especially for cerebrasthenia. In this electrotherapy procedure, the patient held the negative pole, while the physician applied the positive pole to the central nervous system[38] (figs. 8 and 9).

Beard is best remembered for these biological therapies, but a subtext in his works is his attention to and belief in the power of psychological treatment, in particular, the therapeutic relationship for the treatment of neurasthenia. For instance, Beard recognized the importance of "the belief of the power of medicine"—the modern concept of the "placebo effect"—and stated that he had conducted unpublished studies regarding its usefulness in treatment of disease.[39] Since he felt that the mind had power to influence recovery, he emphasized the importance of a positive physician and patient relationship in which hope and careful therapeutic listening were central. Finally, when all else failed, Beard recommended rest, or an extended vacation.

The "rest cure" soon emerged as a leading treatment of neurasthenia. It grew from the concept that the mental and physical work associated with new social, educational, and occupational roles for women led to depletion of nerve force. In *Fat and Blood* (1891), society physician Silas Weir Mitchell proposed his unique approach to "renewing the vitality" of the neurasthenic patient. While Mitchell positioned the rest cure as a biological treatment aimed at increasing the "volume of red corpuscles"[40] and restoring circulation, he in fact

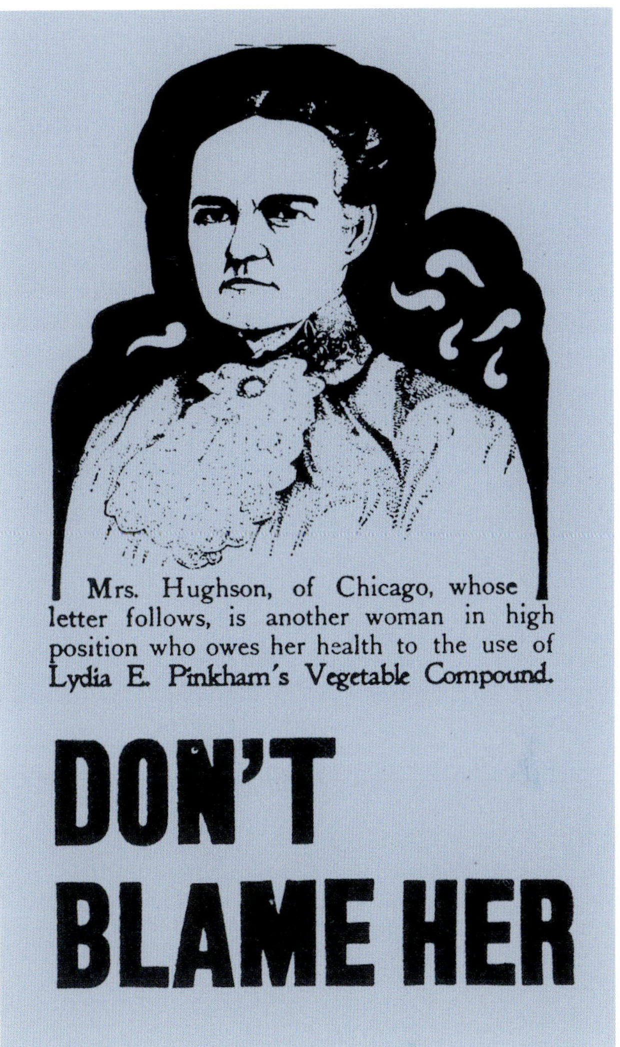

FIG. 5 "Don't Blame Her." Reproduced from Sarah Stage's *Female Complaints: Lydia Pinkham and the Business of Women's Medicine* (New York: W. W. Norton & Co., Inc., 1979). Courtesy of Schlesinger Library.

recognized and attempted to treat the underlying psychological issues involved in some cases of neurasthenia. For instance, he identified the strong interpersonal issues involved in the role of patient when he advocated removal of the patient from her home. "For them there is often no success possible," warned Mitchell, "until we have broken up the whole daily drama of the sick-room, with its little selfishness and its craving for sympathy and indulgence."[41]

Mitchell's prescription was alarmingly confining, for at the beginning the patient was relegated to complete bed rest in a recumbent position for approximately one

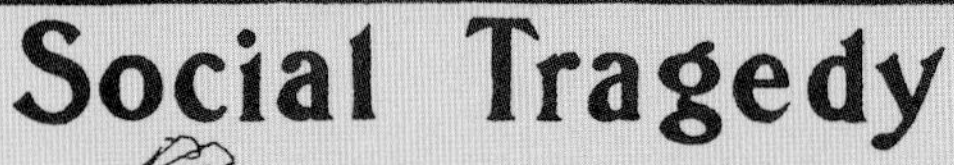

FIG. 6 [*above*] "Social Tragedy," 1896. Courtesy of Schlesinger Library.

FIG. 7 [*right*] "The Studious Girl," 1896. Courtesy of Schlesinger Library.

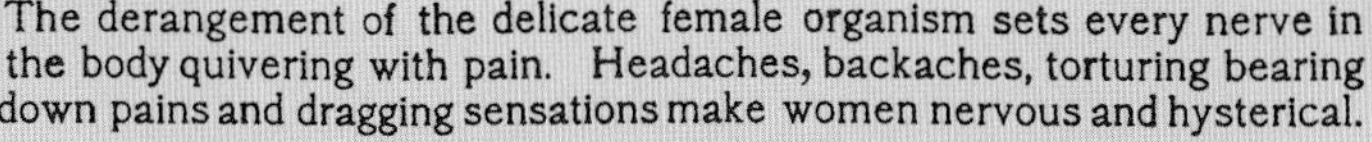

month: "I do not permit the patient to sit up, or to sew or write or read, or to use the hands in any active way except to clean the teeth."[42] The patients were usually fed by a nurse—only milk, initially, but the diet expanded to foods rich in meat, eggs, and butter. In order to stimulate circulation, women were vigorously massaged, often twice a day for an hour. Mitchell also used electricity to give "painless exercise" to the muscles.

Thus, the rest cure has been described in modern terms as "paradoxical psychology." By forcing patients into such a passive position, it led some to abandon the sickness role. The drama of this paternalistic, isolationist approach is luridly depicted by feminist author Charlotte Perkins Gilman in *The Yellow Wallpaper*.[43] Published in book form in 1899, the book is a fictionalized account of Gilman's own experience with neurasthenia and the rest cure under the supervision of "a noted specialist in medical diseases,"[44] most likely S. Weir Mitchell. Years later, describing her reasons for writing the book, Gilman explained that the physician's recommendation to abandon her writing and limit all intellectual pursuits brought her "so near the border line of utter mental ruin" that she wanted to try to save other people from "being driven crazy" by this popular neurasthenia treatment.[45]

Neurasthenia Through a Modern Psychiatric Lens

The question of "nervous exhaustion" in American women remains a timely topic, and the scientific community made unprecedented advances in the last decades of the twentieth century in understanding the interface between gynecology and psychiatry. We are on the brink of a new understanding of the role of the female reproductive cycle in mental illness. Viewed through a modern lens with these findings in mind, how can nineteenth-century neurasthenia be understood?

Careful review of case records reveals that the psychiatric differential diagnosis of neurasthenia clearly included what today are known as affective (mood) disorders. Beard stated that cerebrasthenia included "morbid fears and impulses, depression, insomnia, fulness,

headache, impairment of memory, decline in mental force, and power of control."[46] This description reads like the modern definition of major depression[47] (table 1). Modern epidemiological studies have confirmed that women are 1.7 times more likely than men to suffer from major depression.[48] Furthermore, women are at greatest risk for the onset of major depression during their childbearing years, just as nineteenth-century writers warned.[49]

The causes of increased rates of major depression in American women are complex and multifactorial and include biological, social, and psychological factors.[50] We now know that it is not simply because women have left the traditional domestic sphere to pursue lives in education, business, and medicine that major depression develops. Instead, a seemingly more important psychological risk factor for development of major depression is not whether a woman works outside or inside the home, but whether she feels a sense of loss or conflict or is supported, fulfilled, and inspired by her chosen role.[51]

Recent advances in understanding biological roots of depression in women have focused upon the role of sex steroid hormones in the triggering or exacerbation of illness in a subset of women.[52] Prospective studies have confirmed that a vulnerable group of women exists that is at risk for depressive symptoms at times of hormonal change, such as the premenstruum, the postpartum, and the perimenopause.[53] New biological therapies for these mood episodes associated with hormonal change have included not only traditional antidepressants but also hormonal manipulations such as the suppression of the menstrual cycle, as in treatment-resistant premenstrual syndrome,[54] or treatment of estrogen decline, as in perimenopausal depression.[55]

Nineteenth-century neurasthenia likely included not only major depression but also bipolar affective disorder (commonly known as manic depression). The symptoms of leaden paralysis and severe exhaustion immortalized in the languid and dispirited figures of Thomas Eakins[56] are consistent with the depressive phase of a bipolar illness. Furthermore, the depressive phase of this illness is more common than the manic phase and is associated with protracted debilitation.

FIG. 8 [*right*] "Practical Treatise on Uses of Electricity," 1896. Reproduced from Francis Gosling's *Before Freud: Neurasthenia and the American Medical Community, 1870–1910* (Urbana: University of Illinois Press, 1987).

FIG. 9 [*below*] "The Constant Electric Current, from Our Electric Generator." Constant Current Cure Co., Buffalo, New York.

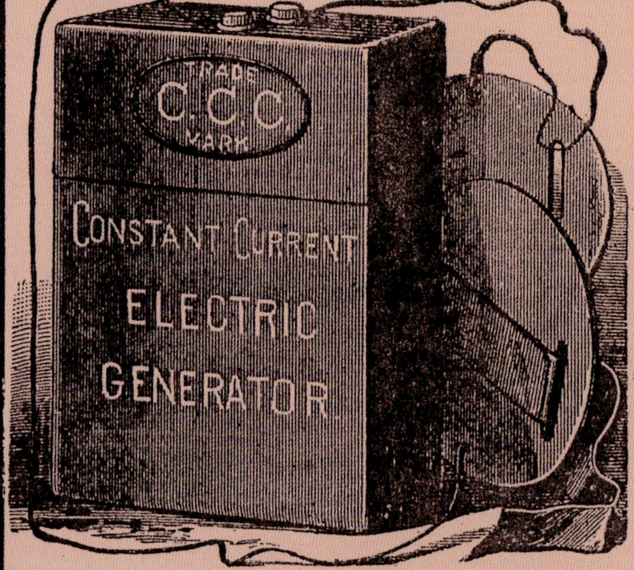

THE CONSTANT ELECTRIC CURRENT,
FROM OUR ELECTRIC GENERATOR,

CURES Headache, Neuralgia, Rheumatism, Pains in the Back, Loins, Limbs, and Kidneys, Extreme Weariness, Nervousness, Incipient Consumption, Piles, Malarial Aches and Pains, Indigestion, Sleeplessness, Debility, Exhaustion, Liver Complaint, and all other diseases requiring the peculiar stimulation afforded by a constant electric current. This gentle stimulation of the affected part induces nutrition in that region, and gives nature the aid required to set all of the repairing agencies actively at work.

This powerful yet simple and compact generator develops a continuous, mild electric current, capable of passing entirely through the human body, affecting every organ, nerve, and tissue, producing marked curative effects.

The current, although so subtile and permeating, is not perceptible to the senses, yet it will operate a galvanometer through a resistance of 5,000 ohms, equal to a telegraph line over 300 miles long.

This truly scientific instrument is indorsed by physicians and electricians, and will cure when all other things fail.

The Constant Current Electric Generator

with full instructions for use, is sent by mail, on receipt of the price, $3.00, or by express, C. O. D., with collection charges added, with the privilege of examination. We guarantee safe delivery of the Generator by mail.
All remittances should be by Postal Money Order, Draft, or Registered Letter.

ONE-HALF SIZE.
PRICE $3.

Fine hard rubber case. Nickel plated binding posts and electrodes. Thoroughly well made and complete. It never gets out of order. ☞ *No acids, no liquids, no trouble.*

CONSTANT CURRENT CURE CO.,
(Incorporated under the laws of the State of New York.) 207 Main St., Buffalo, N. Y.

Indeed, neurasthenics are best remembered for their symptoms of fatigue, but symptoms of agitation, classically seen in the manic phase of bipolar disorder, can also be found in the case reports and descriptions of the illness. For instance, in his case series of five women with neurasthenia published in 1872, T. W. Fisher described one woman who "last night threatened suicide, in a frenzied way, and attempted to jump from the window."[57]

The popularity of sedatives and mood stabilizers, such as lithium, in the treatment of neurasthenia further reinforces this differential diagnosis. Alcohol was another, less well known sedative commonly used in the treatment of "nervous exhaustion." Pinkham's Vegetable Compound was in fact the most alcohol-laden of the patent medicines, as it was composed of 20.6 percent alcohol by volume.[58] Thus, just as bipolar illness today is associated with an increased risk for substance abuse, so was neurasthenia. This relationship between neurasthenia and alcohol is one of the less talked about scripts in the story but one of which Beard himself warned: "Neurasthenia, both of the general form and of the sexual variety, is one of the most frequent of the many exciting causes of inebriety, a nervous disease that may attack those who have never been intemperate."[59]

The relationship between bipolar disorder and postpartum mood disorders is one of the most exciting and productive areas of modern psychiatric and gynecologic research. Recent prospective studies have confirmed that women with a history of bipolar disorder are at significantly increased risk of postpartum depression and psychosis.[60] This finding has led to prophylactic treatment strategies, such as initiating mood stabilizers immediately postpartum, which hold promise for decreasing the morbidity and mortality associated with these serious postpartum psychiatric illnesses.[61]

One of the new areas of research for bipolar and unipolar mood disorders is the use of omega-three fatty acids for both prevention and treatment of depression.[62] It is fascinating to note the importance nineteenth-century practitioners placed on "liberal uses of cod liver oil," since this emulsion is rich in omega-three fatty acids. Similarly, electrical stimulation continues to be refined as an extremely effective method of

TABLE 1

DSM *IV* Diagnostic Criteria for *Major Depressive Episode*

Five (or more) of the following symptoms have been present during the same 2-week period and represent a change from previous functioning; at least one of the symptoms is either (1) depressed mood or (2) loss of interest or pleasure.

Note: Do not include symptoms that are clearly due to a general medical condition, or mood-incongruent delusions or hallucinations.

1. depressed mood most of the day, nearly every day, as indicated by either subjective report (e.g., feels sad or empty) or observation made by others (e.g., appears tearful)
2. markedly diminished interest or pleasure in all, or almost all, activities most of the day, nearly every day
3. significant weight loss when not dieting, . . . or decrease or increase in appetite nearly every day
4. insomnia or hypersomnia nearly every day
5. psychomotor agitation or retardation nearly every day
6. fatigue or loss of energy nearly every day
7. feelings of worthlessness or excessive or inappropriate guilt nearly every day
8. diminished ability to think or concentrate, or indecisiveness, nearly every day
9. recurrent thoughts of death (not just fear of dying), recurrent suicidal ideation without a specific plan, or a suicide attempt or a specific plan for committing suicide

Reprinted from the *American Psychiatric Association Diagnostic and Statistical Manual of Mental Disorders*, 4th ed. (Washington, D.C.: American Psychiatric Association, 1994), 327.

obsessive-compulsive disorder, or OCD (table 3).
Fisher described a woman likely tormented with OCD
when he reported her "mania for precise adjustment of
certain things. Exhausts herself rearranging clothing in
closets and dishes on shelves from a weak fear that they
will fall on the floor if left alone."[64] Modern psychiatric
research has found that anxiety disorders in women are
indeed influenced by the reproductive cycle; women
with a history of OCD, for instance, experience more
symptoms at times of hormonal change, such as the
premenstruum and postpartum.[65]

Neurasthenia in nineteenth-century women most
likely encompassed the modern notion of eating disorders as well. Mitchell wrote in the introduction to *Fat
and Blood* that his cure came from his clinical experience
with "that large group of nervous women, who as a rule,
are thin and lack blood."[66] He hypothesized that fat was
necessary for the formation of red blood cells, and so a
diet rich in fat was necessary for restoration of health.
He spoke of the precipitating psychological stress, or
the medical illness with attendant weight loss, that then
starts a cycle of weight loss and debility. When Cleaves
described a young woman patient who refused to
eat, engaged in frequent vomiting, and presented as
extremely thin, she provided a vision of the modern
purging subtype of anorexia nervosa. After disengaging
the patient from her family and slowly feeding her,
Cleaves actually accomplished the goal set out in the
American Psychiatric Association (APA) guidelines
for weight gain in anorexia nervosa: two pounds per
week.[67] Cleaves was hopeful that when her patient
regained enough weight, her menstrual cycle would
return, a result that modern psychiatric and gynecological research has since documented.

Other possible medical causes of neurasthenia that
are now known to be more common in women include
endocrinopathies such as thyroid disease and autoim-
mune illnesses such as multiple sclerosis and systemic
lupus erythematosis. Furthermore, the modern medical
mysteries chronic fatigue syndrome and fibromyalgia
are very similar to neurasthenia.[68] Like neurasthenia,
these illnesses include vague symptoms of exhaustion,
sleep disturbance, pain, and neuropsychiatric complaints. At present, both illnesses lack a unifying,

treating mood disorders, and the modern transmag-
netic cranial stimulation procedure is reminiscent of
Beard's central galvanization.[63]

The modern diagnostic criteria for generalized
anxiety disorder bear a striking resemblance to descriptions of nervous exhaustion (table 2). Another
important, yet less recognized historical detail is
that neurasthenia included what today is known as

clear physiological explanation, and no agreed-upon laboratory abnormalities or diagnostic tests prove the existence of either chronic fatigue syndrome or fibromyalgia.[69] As in the treatment of neurasthenia, diet, exercise, and psychotherapy have all been helpful in decreasing symptoms and restoring functioning.[70]

In conclusion, neurasthenia in nineteenth-century American women was an illness with unique social and cultural nuances and medical complexities. When viewed with a modern lens, it clearly encompassed what today are recognized as a variety of medical and psychiatric disorders that are known to be more common in women. For American women on the verge of a new century, the illness came to represent both the tensions and the promise of the coming age. By the early 1900s, many extraordinary changes occurred in women's roles and in the scientific knowledge of the safety of higher education for women and work outside the home. The rise of psychoanalysis expanded the formulation of the mind-body connection, and, over time, the popularity of the diagnosis of neurasthenia began to fade. As one medical writer wrote while in the process of deconstructing the disease, "I must confess that I may be charged with dealing disrespectfully with our one great national malady."[71]

Notes

The author wishes to acknowledge the scholarship of Sarah Stage, who uncovered several of the popular neurasthenia treatment advertisements reprinted here while researching her book *Female Complaints: Lydia Pinkham and the Business of Women's Medicine*. Her book, an invaluable contribution to the history of women and medicine, inspired the curators to search for other advertisements for the exhibition. Many thanks to Jacalyn Bloom, Linda Morrison, and the Schlesinger Library at Harvard University for locating these additional images and permitting us to reprint them, and to Jeanie Lawrence for expertly overseeing the details of this project. Finally, thanks to Dr. Claire Perry for her enthusiasm and vision, which enabled us to blend the worlds of art and medicine and create *Women on the Verge*.

1. For a comprehensive review of the unique American experience of neurasthenia, see Francis G. Gosling, *Before Freud: Neurasthenia and the American Medical Community, 1870–1910* (Urbana: University of Illinois Press, 1987); Tom Lutz, *American Nervousness, 1903: An Anecdotal History* (Ithaca, NY: Cornell

TABLE 3

DSM *IV Diagnostic Criteria for Obsessive-Compulsive Disorder*

A. Either obsessions or compulsions:
Obsessions defined by (1), (2), (3), and (4):

1. recurrent and persistent thoughts, impulses, or images that are experienced, at some time during the disturbance, as intrusive and inappropriate, and cause marked anxiety or distress

2. the thoughts, impulses, or images are not simply excessive worries about real-life problems

3. the person attempts to ignore or suppress the thoughts, impulses, or images, or to neutralize them with another thought or action

4. the person recognizes that the obsessional thoughts, impulses, or images are from his or her own mind

Compulsions as defined by (1) and (2):

1. repetitive behaviors (e.g., hand washing, ordering, checking) or mental acts (e.g., praying, counting, repeating words silently) the person feels driven to perform in response to an obsession, or according to rules that must be rigidly applied

2. the behaviors or mental acts are aimed at preventing or reducing distress or preventing some dreaded event or situation; however, these behaviors or mental acts either are not connected in a realistic way with what they are designed to neutralize or prevent, or are clearly excessive

B. At some point during the course of the disorder, the person has recognized that the obsessions or compulsions are excessive or unreasonable

C. The obsessions or compulsions cause marked distress, are time consuming (take more than 1 hour a day), or significantly interfere with the person's normal routine, occupational (or academic) functioning, or usual social activities or relationships

Reprinted from the *American Psychiatric Association Diagnostic and Statistical Manual of Mental Disorders*, 4th ed. (Washington, D.C.: American Psychiatric Association, 1994), 422–23.

University Press, 1991); and *Cultures of Neurasthenia from Beard to the First World War*, ed. Marijke Gijswijt-Hofstra and Roy Porter (Amsterdam: Rodopi, 2001), 51–76.

2. The purpose of this paper and the exhibition *Women on the Verge* has been to highlight the unique female representations of neurasthenia in art and culture in nineteenth-century America. It is important to note, however, that while neurasthenia was described as more common in women than in men, statistics do not support such a sex difference. See Gosling, *Before Freud*, 34–35.

3. George M. Beard, "Neurasthenia, or Nervous Exhaustion," *Boston Medical and Surgical Journal* 89 (1869): 217–21.

4. Ibid., 218.

5. George M. Beard, *Sexual Neurasthenia (Nervous Exhaustion): Its Hygiene, Causes, Symptoms, and Treatment* (New York: E. B. Treat, 1884), 43.

6. George M. Beard, *American Nervousness: Its Causes and Consequences* (New York: G. P. Putnam's Sons, 1881), 20.

7. Ibid., 207.

8. Ibid., 184–86.

9. Ibid., 26. For a discussion of the status and gender issues involved in the differential diagnosis and treatment of neurasthenia, see Barbara Sicherman, "The Uses of a Diagnosis: Doctors, Patients, and Neurasthenia," *Journal of the History of Medicine* 32 (1977): 33–45.

10. Quoted in Ann Douglas Wood, "'The Fashionable Diseases': Women's Complaints and Their Treatment in Nineteenth-Century America," *Journal of Nervous and Mental Disease* 7 (1880): 1–16. Reprinted in *Journal of Interdisciplinary History* 4 (Summer 1973): 29.

11. James S. Jewell, "The Varieties and Causes of Neurasthenia," *The Journal of Nervous and Mental Disease* 7 (1880): 1–16.

12. See Catherine M. Scholten, "'On the importance of the Obstetrick Art': Changing Customs of Childbirth in America, 1760 to 1825," in *History of Women in the United States*, ed. Nancy F. Cott (Munich: K. G. Saur, 1993), 3–22.

13. See Frances E. Kobrin, "The American Midwife Controversy: A Crisis of Professionalization," in Cott, *History of Women*, 278–91; Judy Barrett Litoff, "Forgotten Women: American Midwives at the Turn of the Twentieth Century," in Cott, *History of Women*, 292–308; Judith Walzer Leavitt, "Science Enters the Birthing Room: Obstetrics in America since the Eighteenth Century," in Cott, *History of Women*, 324–47; and Janet Carlisle Bogan, "Childbirth in America, 1650–1990," in *Women, Health, and Medicine in America: A Historical Handbook*, ed. Rima D. Apple (New York: Garland Publishing, Inc., 1990), 101–20.

14. See Regina Markell Morantz, "Making Women Modern: Middle-Class Women and Health Reform in Nineteenth-Century America," in Cott, *History of Women*, 156–73.

15. See Judith Walzer Leavitt, "Under the Shadow of Maternity: American Women's Responses to Death and Debility Fears in Nineteenth-Century Childbirth," in Cott, *History of Women*, 252–77.

16. Beard, *American Nervousness*, 77.

17. Quoted in Barbara Ehrenreich and Deirdre English, *For Her Own Good: 150 Years of the Experts' Advice to Women* (New York: Doubleday, 1978), 110.

18. Beard, *American Nervousness*, 76.

19. See John S. Haller, "From Maidenhood to Menopause: Sex Education for Women in Victorian America," in Cott, *History of Women*, 174–94.

20. Beard explicitly stated that "the mental activity of women" was one of five primary causes of neurasthenia in *American Nervousness*, 96.

21. Margaret A. Cleaves, "Neurasthenia and Its Relation to Diseases of Women," *Transactions of the Iowa State Medical Association* 9 (1886): 166–67.

22. Quoted in Carroll Smith-Rosenberg and Charles Rosenberg, "The Female Animal: Medical and Biological Views of Woman and Her Role in Nineteenth-Century America," in Cott, *History of Women*, 49.

23. Leavitt, "Shadow of Maternity," in Cott, *History of Women*, 255.

24. Edward H. Clarke, *Sex in Education, or, a Fair Chance for the Girls* (Boston: J. R. Osgood, 1873).

25. John Dewy, "Health and Sex in Higher Education," *Popular Science Monthly* 28 (1889): 606.

26. Not all nineteenth-century physicians subscribed to the idea that study led to neurasthenia in women. See Anita Claire Fellman and Michael Fellman, *Making Sense of Self: Medical Advice Literature in Late Nineteenth-Century America* (Philadelphia: University of Pennsylvania Press, 1981), 68–69.

27. Beard, *Sexual Neurasthenia*, 26.

28. See Sarah Stage, *Female Complaints: Lydia Pinkham and the Business of Women's Medicine* (New York: W. W. Norton & Co., Inc., 1979), 78–79.

29. Leavitt, "Shadow of Maternity," in Cott, *History of Women*, 260.

30. Stage, 79.

31. Ehrenreich and English, *For Her Own Good*, 108–10.

32. See Robin M. Haller and John S. Haller, Jr., *The Physician and Sexuality in Nineteenth-Century America* (Urbana: University of Illinois Press, 1974), 162–74.

33. Frances Willard quoted in Richard Leeman, ed., *"Do Everything Reform": The Oratory of Frances Willard* (New York: Greenwood Press, 1992), 157.

34. Vern Bullough and Martha Voght, "Women, Menstruation, and Nineteenth-Century Medicine," in Cott, *History of Women*, 230–39.

35. See G. J. Barker-Benfield, *The Horrors of the Half-Known Life* (New York: Harper & Row, 1976); Gosling, *Before Freud*, 57–62; Ehrenreich and English, *For Her Own Good*, 120–25;

Judith M. Roy, "Surgical Gynecology," in Apple, *Women, Health, and Medicine in America*, 173–91.

36. For a detailed history of the Lydia Pinkham Company, see Stage, *Female Complaints*.

37. John Stea, "Remedies for Society's Debilities: Medicines for Neurasthenia in Victorian America," *New York State Journal of Medicine* 93 (1993): 120–27. See Gosling, *Before Freud*, 108–43.

38. Gosling, 123–24.

39. Beard, *Sexual Neurasthenia*, 221.

40. S. Weir Mitchell, *Fat and Blood: An Essay on the Treatment of Certain Forms of Neurasthenia and Hysteria* (London: J. B. Lippincott & Co., 1891), 24.

41. Ibid., 49.

42. Ibid., 58.

43. Charlotte Perkins (Stetson) Gilman, *The Yellow Wallpaper*, 1899. Reprinted with an afterword by Elaine R. Hedges (New York: The Feminist Press, 1973).

44. Charlotte Perkins Gilman, "Why I Wrote the Yellow Wall-paper," *The Forerunner* 4 (October 1913): 271.

45. Ibid.

46. Beard, *Sexual Neurasthenia*, 47.

47. *American Psychiatric Association Diagnostic and Statistical Manual of Mental Disorders*, 4th ed. (Washington, D.C.: American Psychiatric Association, 1994).

48. See Ronald Kessler, "Gender Differences in the Prevalence and Correlates of Mood Disorders in the General Population," in *Mood Disorders in Women*, ed. Meir Steiner, Kimberly Yonkers, and Elias Eriksson (London: Martin Dunitz, 2000), 15–33.

49. See Kathleen Merikangas, "Epidemiology of Mood Disorders in Women," in Steiner, Yonkers, and Eriksson, *Mood Disorders in Women*, 1–14.

50. For an excellent review, see Susan Nolan Hoeksema, "Epidemiology and Theories of Gender Differences in Unipolar Depression," in *Gender and Psychopathology*, ed. Mary V. Seeman (Washington, D.C.: American Psychiatric Press, Inc., 1995), 63–87.

51. See Natalie Rasgon, Michael McGuire, and Alfonso Troisi, "Evolutionary Concepts of Gender Differences in Depressive Disorders," in Steiner, Yonkers, and Eriksson, *Mood Disorders in Women*, 35–45.

52. Katherine Williams and Regina Casper, "Reproduction and Its Psychopathology," in *Women, Health and Hormones*, ed. Regina Casper (Cambridge, Eng.: Cambridge University Press, 1998), 14–35.

53. A. J. Rapkin, J. A. Mikacich, B. Moatakef-Imani, and N. L. Rasgon, "The Clinical Nature and Diagnosis of Premenstrual, Postpartum and Perimenopausal Affective Disorders,"

Current Psychiatry Report 4 (2002): 419–28; and H. Joffe and L. S. Cohen, "Estrogen, Serotonin, and Mood Disorders: Where Is the Therapeutic Bridge?" *Biological Psychiatry* 44 (1998): 330–40.

54. Williams and Casper, 20.

55. N. L. Rasgon, L. L. Altshuler, L. A. Fairbanks, et al., "Estrogen Replacement Therapy in the Treatment of Major Depressive Disorder in Perimenopausal Women," *Journal of Clinical Psychiatry* 63, suppl. 7 (2002): 45–48.

56. See Kathleen Spies's essay in this catalogue, 37–51.

57. T. W. Fisher, "Neurasthenia," *Boston Medical and Surgical Journal* 9 (1872): 69.

58. Haller and Haller, 287–90.

59. Beard, *Sexual Neurasthenia*, 44.

60. Linda H. Chaudron and Ronald W. Pies, "The Relationship Between Postpartum Psychosis and Bipolar Disorder: A Review," *Journal of Clinical Psychiatry* 64 (2003): 1284–90.

61. See Donna Stewart, "Prophylactic Lithium in Postpartum Affective Psychosis," *Journal of Nervous Mental Disorders* 76 (1988): 486–89; and D. E. Stewart, J. L. Klompenhouwer, R. E. Kendell, et al., "Prophylactic Lithium in Puerperal Psychosis: The Experience of Three Centres," *British Journal of Psychiatry* 158 (1991): 393–97.

62. For a review, see "Brain Stimulation Methods in the Treatment of Affective Disorders," *CNS Spectrums* 8, ed. Thomas E. Schlaepfer, 8 (July 2003).

63. Ibid.

64. Fisher, 70.

65. Katherine Williams and Lorin Koran, "Obsessive-Compulsive Disorder in Pregnancy, the Premenstrum and Postpartum," *Journal of Clinical Psychiatry* 58 (1997): 330–34.

66. Mitchell, 9.

67. American Psychiatric Association, "Practice Guidelines for Eating Disorders," *American Journal of Psychiatry* 150 (1993): 212–20.

68. See Susan E. Abbey and Paul E. Garfinkel, "Neurasthenia and Chronic Fatigue Syndrome: The Role of Culture in the Making of a Diagnosis," *American Journal of Psychiatry* 148 (1991): 1638–46.

69. M. B. Yunus, "Gender Differences in Fibromyalgia and Other Related Syndromes," *Journal of Gender-Specific Medicine* 5 (2002): 43–47.

70. B. Evengard and N. Klimas, "Chronic Fatigue Syndrome: Probable Pathogenesis and Possible Treatments," *Drugs* 62 (2002): 2433–46.

71. Charles L. Dana, "The Partial Passing of Neurasthenia," *Boston Medical and Surgical Journal* 150 (1904): 339–44.

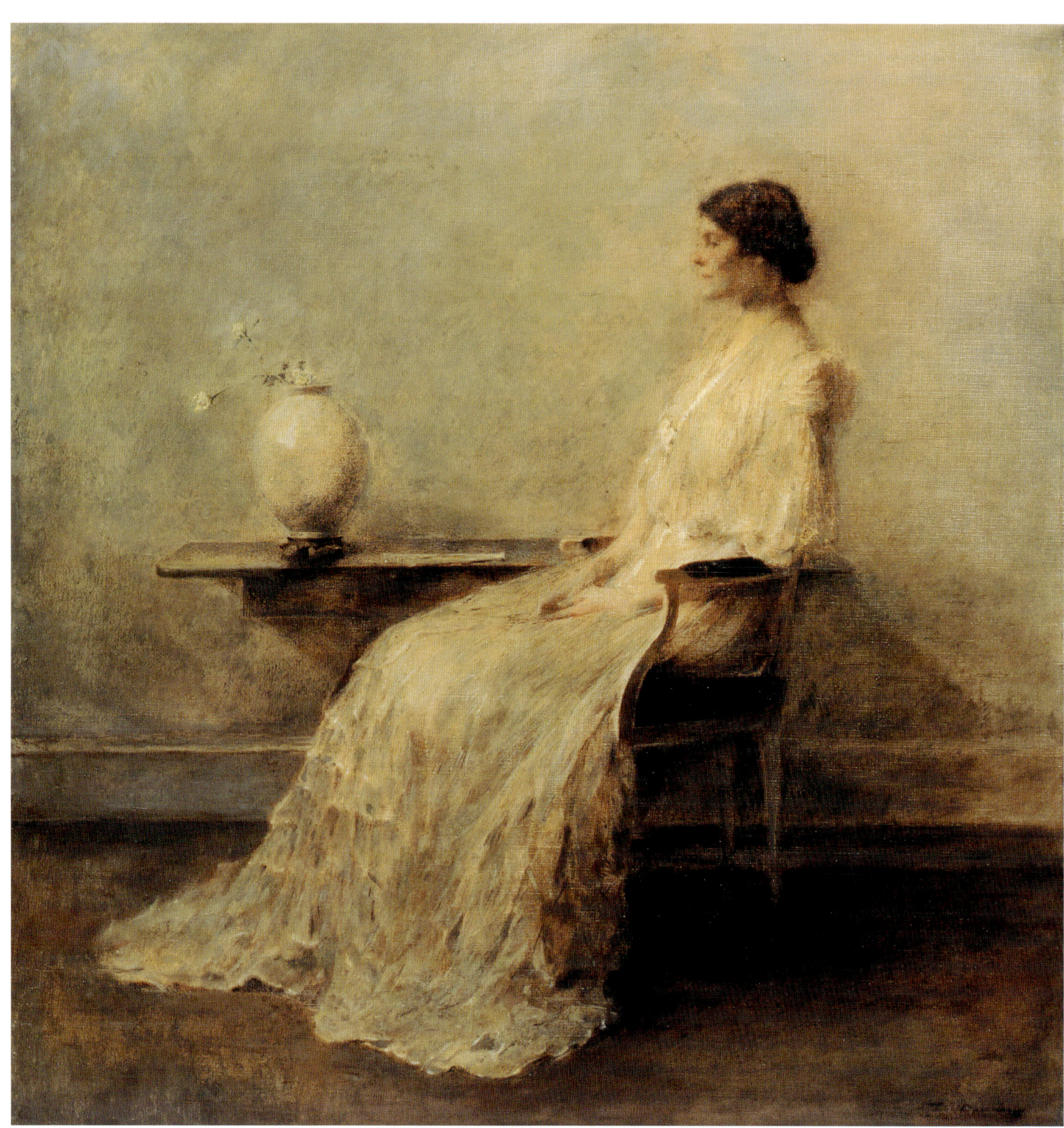

ZACHARY ROSS

REST FOR THE WEARY

AMERICAN NERVOUSNESS
AND THE AESTHETICS OF REPOSE

Paintings of weary women relaxing in interior settings, such as Thomas Wilmer Dewing's *Lady in White (No. 2)*, abounded in America's Gilded Age (fig. 10). While much has been written in recent years to explain the development of the woman-in-interior motif, or what we might call the "Woman at Home," in the present essay I attempt to add to this chorus by relating the popularity of the genre to society's urgent quest for rest and repose.[1] Through their emphasis on decorative harmony and bodily and mental relaxation, paintings such as *Lady in White* functioned phenomenologically to help induce a state of inward repose, a key therapeutic ideal eagerly sought by both male and female viewers.[2] Emblematic of the Woman at Home, Dewing's *Lady in White* bears a tired, almost emotionless expression. Seated before a simple table and portrayed in profile, she stares passively in the direction of the flower vase that rests at the end of the table, acknowledging neither the viewer nor her spare surroundings. She is alone and lost in a private moment of passive introspection, her body relaxed and her hands resting comfortably in her lap. Her isolation within the composition implies a meditative withdrawal from affairs of the present. This sense of psychic distance is reinforced

by the translucent veil of green and gold paint that suffuses the entirety of the picture plane. The paint is so thinly applied in a flickering, stippled technique as to suggest that the entire painting is nothing more than an apparition. The total effect of Dewing's painting is that the woman appears absorbed into an oceanic, spiritual ether, a realm of mental calm and tranquility. The painting's anonymous title establishes that it is not a portrait, and that we, too, are meant to interpret it passively, to receive through aesthetic contemplation its message of physical and emotional repose.

Repose was a major preoccupation of the Gilded Age, emerging as a main prescription for alleviating the stress of modern life. As the rationalization of the business world invaded the domestic sphere, Americans increasingly struggled to "keep up," to be "on time," to not be left behind by the changes being made swiftly to American civilization.[3] The psychological dislocation and anxiety Americans experienced as a result of the perceived "overcivilization" of society—driven by such technological innovations as steam power, the railroad,

FIG. 10 [*facing*] Thomas Wilmer Dewing,
Lady in White (No. 2.), c. 1910. Oil on canvas, 22⅜ × 21⅜ in.
Smithsonian American Art Museum. Gift of John Gellatly.

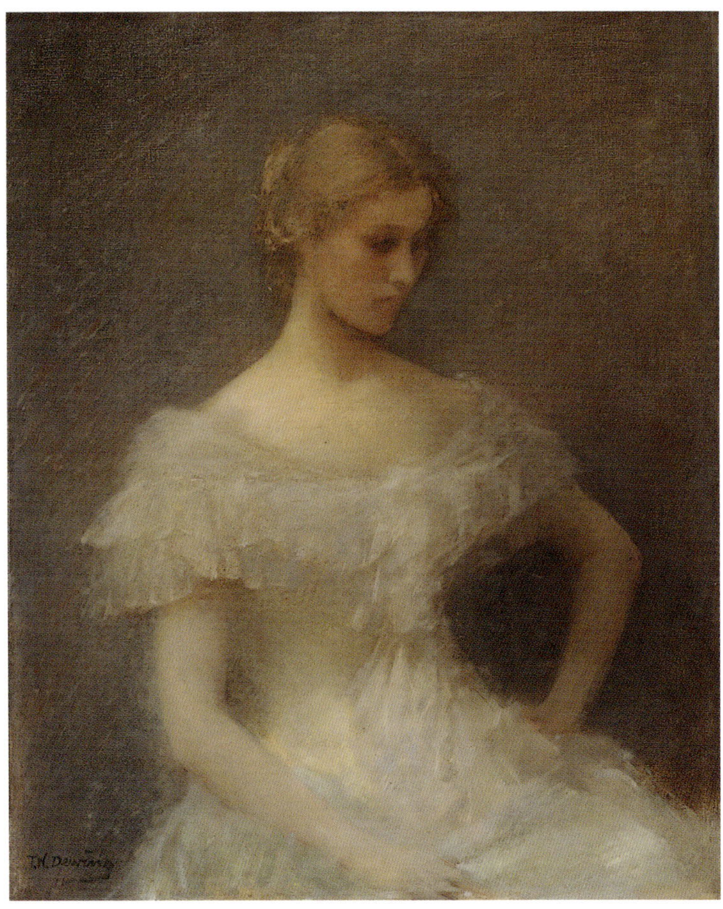

FIG. 11 Thomas Wilmer Dewing, *Young Girl Seated*, 1896. Oil on canvas, 20⅛ × 18⅛ in. Smithsonian American Art Museum. Gift of John Gellatly.

and the telegraph, and exacerbated by the threat of immigration—manifested themselves in the newly identified medical condition of neurasthenia. As set forth by the neurologist George Beard in his famous *American Nervousness: Its Causes and Consequences*, neurasthenia was responsible for a wide variety of chronic health problems arising from an overstressed nervous system.[4] Overworked nerves ultimately led to a nervous breakdown or, in the language of the time, "nervous prostration." In Beard's estimation, people of "refined sensibilities," such as business leaders, writers, artists, and others of the "higher orders" of society who endured intense mental and emotional stresses, were particularly likely to suffer from neurasthenia because they were more apt to "overdraw" their supply of nervous energy. Neurasthenia, known more popularly as "nervousness," "Americanitis," or even just "that tired

feeling," became the most widely diagnosed neurological illness of the Gilded Age. Beard's views on neurasthenia resonated with a population concerned not only with its health and ability to adapt to modern society, but also with securing its place in the middle and upper reaches of the social ladder. This had particular significance among the upper classes of New England —the epicenter of nervousness, according to Beard— whose cultural hegemony was most at risk during this period. Within these circles, nervousness became a social-Darwinian signifier of one's social respectability: for men, the illness confirmed their position as masters of the emergent capitalist order, while for women it served as a sign of intellectual refinement and eminence in polite society.[5]

The rise in popularity of the Woman at Home genre coincided with the ascendance of nervousness in the American consciousness. The Woman at Home was a component of the therapeutic discourse of the age, as it acted as an agent against nervousness. How paintings of women in repose functioned within this discourse can best be seen through the study of the artist who developed the genre's therapeutic potential to its fullest, Thomas Wilmer Dewing.[6] Combining pictorial strategies from a variety of sources, including the art of Whistler, Vermeer, Japanese ukiyo-e master Kitagawa Utamaro, and Edgar Degas,[7] Dewing's pictures, particularly those of his later career, directly engage contemporary beliefs about both the therapeutic value of art and the role of self-determined physical and emotional relaxation in overcoming nervousness.[8] Dewing's works were lauded by critics of the period, who considered them a most rarefied and modern corpus of paintings. (One critic asserted that "a key is needed to appreciate them which some critics and many gallery visitors do not possess.")[9] His paintings stood apart from his contemporaries in the evocation of repose, and they were appreciated by just a handful of elite collectors, the foremost among them being the chronically neurasthenic railroad industrialist and aesthete, Charles Lang Freer. The purity of Dewing's evocation of repose eased the nervous tensions of collectors like Freer, for whom Dewing's paintings represented the mind transcended from the stresses of modern life.[10]

Ideas about nervousness are deeply embedded in Dewing's paintings. The tired expression, attenuated figure, and languid countenance of Dewing's exemplary *Lady in White* and the air of hushed, almost melancholy stillness of the environment in which she sits certainly have resonance with the archetypically weary and reticent sufferer of neurasthenia. Similarly, a palpable feeling of *tristesse* emanates from Dewing's *Young Girl Seated* (fig. 11), who casts her dark, weary eyes downward in a moment of introspection. The painting sounds a moody note by casting the girl's face in shadow, which is all the more emphasized by the diaphanous brilliance of the young woman's dress that Dewing paints in gauzy layers of white. This girl is furthermore shown alone against a dark, formless backdrop, adding to the sense of psychic isolation and withdrawal. She seems a potential candidate for Philadelphia neurologist S. Weir Mitchell's oppressive "rest cure," the infamous medical prescription for female neurasthenics that prescribed six to eight weeks of bed rest, seclusion, and mental inactivity.[11]

But as tempting as it may be to read these and other pictures of genteel women as sufferers of nervousness in need of medical attention, in fact one finds few unambiguous representations of neurasthenic women in American art.[12] For despite neurasthenia's "fashionable" appeal, a number of negative connotations accreted to the female neurasthenic, who came to be regarded by many as an ignoble home-wrecking force, selfish in her "morbid introspection" and need for attention, and as a drain on the household's spirits.[13] She also became the subject of ridicule in fiction and the theater, mocked for her trifling worries and self-indulgent behavior[14] (fig. 12). Furthermore, in an age when the ugly scourge of invalidism was widespread and touched nearly every household at one time or another, high art, with its traditional beautifying and refining mission, generally elided overt depictions of nervous women or women under treatment for nervousness.[15] For example, the women in Dewing's *Young Girl Seated* and Henry Ossawa Tanner's *Portrait of the Artist's Wife* (fig. 13), with their downcast gazes suggesting an air of melancholy and fatigue, nevertheless command a certain dignity in their relaxed posture and are far from suggesting an

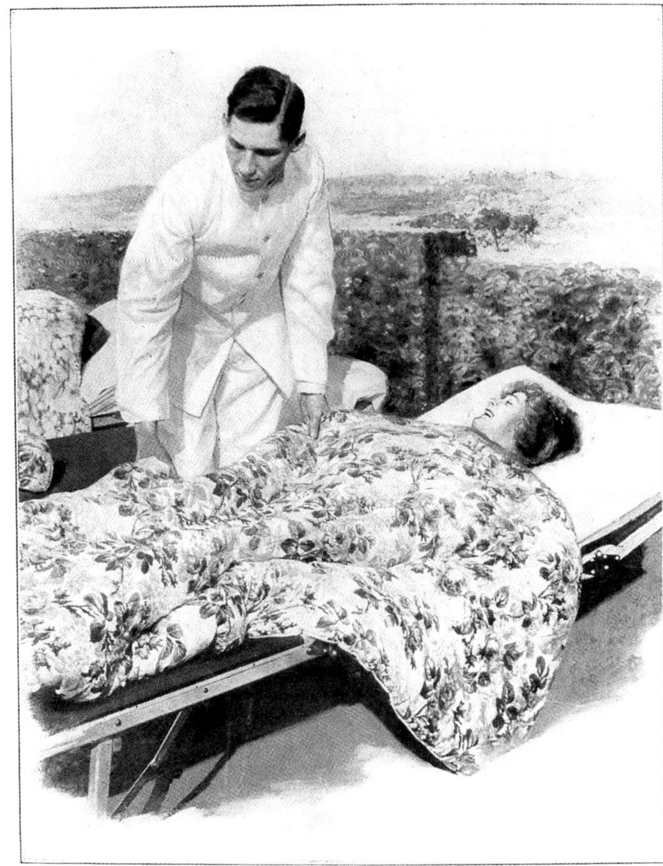

FIG. 12 Frontispiece from Ruth McEnery Stuart, *The Cocoon: A Rest-Cure Comedy*, 1915. New York: Hearst's International Library Company. Photo Courtesy of Helga Studios.

incapacitated state of nervous prostration. While these women evince recognizable signs of nervousness—weary expressions, pale complexions, attenuated figures, and averted eyes—they are not the subjects of the rest cure, which in its strict emphasis on inactivity was essentially an enforced invalidism. Rather, artists like Dewing, while visually acknowledging the Woman at Home's "natural" predisposition toward nervousness, instead developed an ideal type that both acknowledged and emphasized the subjects' social refinement as well as their attainment of physical and mental relaxation. The Woman at Home, in this therapeutic construct, is in the process of *becoming*: on the verge of neurasthenia, she achieves repose and eases her psychic tensions.

Artists, critics, and collectors alike believed that the

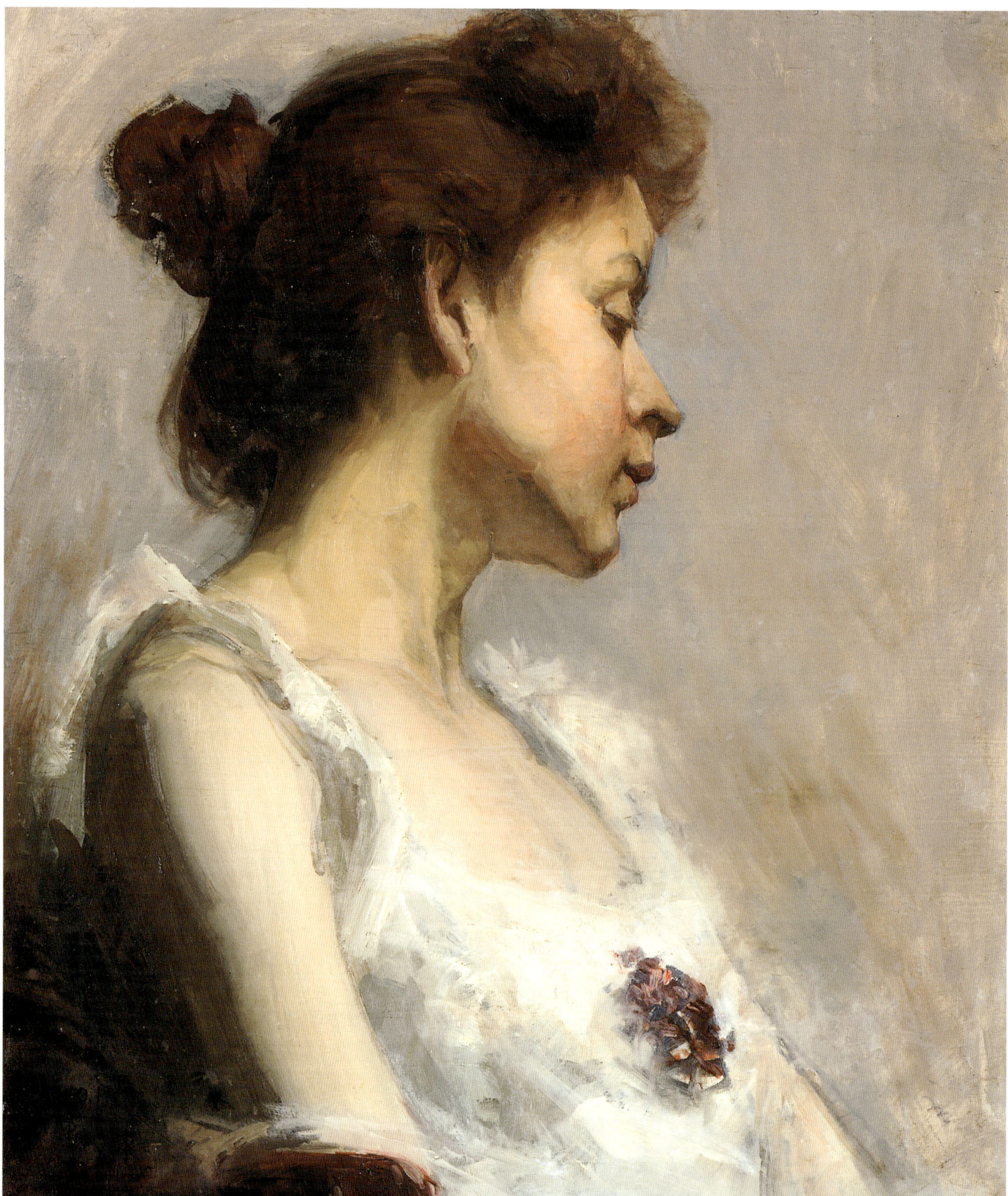

experience of a "pure" work of art served a therapeutic function by acting "directly on the nerves, the chief possession, or affliction, of these restless modern days."[16] In this formulation, art provided the viewer with a conduit to a spiritualized realm of rest and relaxation that helped heal frayed and damaged nerves.[17] Paintings of the Woman at Home—devoid of narrative, their emphasis instead on beauty and the viewer's aesthetic contemplation—fit the ideal of the therapeutic work of art. Dewing's *Lady in White*, sitting passively and suffused in an aestheticized, spiritual ether brimming with potential energy, transcends the worries of the modern world and conveys a mood of pure relaxation. This is the key idea behind Dewing's painting. The *Lady in White*'s transformation from nervous wreck to model of relaxation serves as an exemplar for the viewer, who achieves repose through the contemplation of the pure work of art.[18]

At this point one may ask why Dewing and other artists turned almost exclusively to women and not men in these interior-genre paintings; that is, why is there not an analogous Man at Home? Due to their associations with the strenuous mental activity of the business world and not with the domestic ideal of the home, men were inadequate symbols to convey the ideal of relaxation and repose. Men's symbolic potential for easing the tensions of nervousness lay in physical action. A more manly prescription for neurasthenia than the rest cure was strenuous exercise and outdoor activity; Winslow Homer, for example, painted scenes of male action and the rugged New England outdoors that helped rejuvenate world-weary male viewers.[19] Although many new roles were available to women in this period, many of which treaded upon the ground of traditional male activities, women's genteel associations with purity, taste, refinement, and the domestic sphere were best suited to represent repose, the ideal anodyne to the nerve-wracking chaos of modern life.[20]

In constructing the ideal prototype of the Woman at Home, artists like Dewing engaged the discourse of the popular psychology of mind cure.[21] Reeling from the injurious "wear and tear" (a term coined by S. Weir Mitchell) to their nerves and fearful of lapsing into nervousness, Americans were urged to heed the "gospel of rest" and to disengage themselves from the tumult of the modern world.[22] As the nineteenth century drew to a close, oppressive measures such as Mitchell's rest cure gave way to more positive, self-directed remedies in the form of "New Thought," or what William James called the "mind-cure movement."[23] A form of therapy designed to curtail the depletion of personal energies resulting from overexcitement of the nerves, mind cure asserted a fundamental interconnectedness of mind and body, which supported the notion that mental forces were the preeminent determiners of health. Mental hygienists widely agreed that rest was required in order to maintain control of the emotions, as a lack of emotional control was the most commonly identified cause of neurasthenia.[24] Mind-cure practice involved achieving both physical and mental relaxation, opening the mind to an abundant reservoir of cosmic energy that replenished the weary nervous system and healed damaged nerves. Mind cure thus promised a means of autonomously achieving health through "right thinking" and self-control. As such, mind-cure ideology was a modern manifestation of the Protestant ethos of self-discipline and moral rectitude, and it had particular appeal among the cultural elite in New England and those who aspired to its old-world, patrician ideals, including artists like Dewing and the captains of industry who were their greatest patrons.

Aimed at both men and women, a proliferation of mind-cure advice books and magazines capitalizing on the furor over nervousness offered lessons on how to control one's emotions and calm one's nerves (fig. 14). As one author put it, "Self-control is the crying need of the hour."[25] Among the most popular of these publications was Annie Payson Call's *Power Through Repose*, which followed the standard mind-cure prescription for psychic renewal through the establishment of an equilibrium between body and mind.[26] Asserting that tensions in the body were related to stresses in the mind, Call instructed her readers to cultivate the body's ability to relax and move effortlessly. With the body

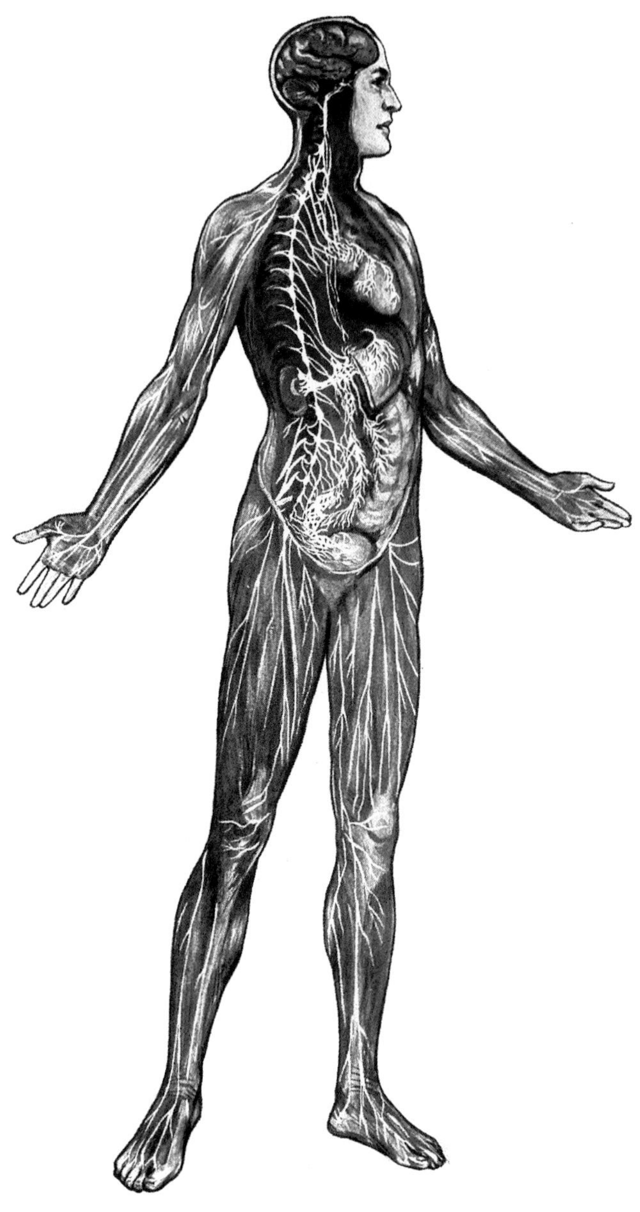

FIG. 14 Frontispiece from William S. Sadler, *Worry and Nervousness: The Science of Self-Mastery*, 1914. Chicago: A. C. McClurg & Co. Photo Courtesy of Helga Studios.

performing efficiently so that a minimum of nervous force was expended, the mind was free to keep one's emotions in a healthy, balanced state. From this state of repose came power.

> Whenever the brain alone is used in thinking, or in receiving and taking note of impressions through either of the senses, new power comes as we gain freedom from all misdirected force, and with muscles in repose leave the brain to quietly do its work without useless strain of any kind.[27]

In order to attain repose, "The first care should be to gain quiet, as through repose of mind and body we cultivate the power to 'erase all previous impressions.'"[28] This explains the atmosphere of silence of Dewing's *Lady in White* and the blank, almost emotionless look on the woman's face: free from distractions and with her mind clear, the path is open to healthful, unworried thought, not the morbid introspection of the neurasthenic.

Echoing beliefs about the transformative power of art shared by their artist contemporaries, many doctors and mind-curists advocated mental recreation as a potent means of repose, which could be achieved through such genteel channels as the collecting and contemplation of art objects, rare books and prints, china, and furniture.[29] In keeping with this idea, Dewing's *Lady in White* eases into her repose while contemplating the fine flower vase before her. Under the rubric of mind cure, fantasy and introspection were no longer threatening to one's health, but instead were constructive endeavors that replenished and even increased one's psychic resources. This helps to explain the large number of paintings of the period titled *Reverie*—a particularly common variant of the Woman at Home—by such artists as Dewing, Edmund Tarbell, Alice Pike Barney, Robert Frederick Blum, and Irving Ramsay Wiles, among many others. These paintings of women lost in aesthetic contemplation and playful reverie embody the mind-cure ideal of renewed power through mental recreation, and they also provide positive visual cues for viewers to achieve their own aesthetic release from battered nerves through the contemplation of the work of art.

Mind-curists like Call offered programmatic methods of nerve-force conservation with a strong moral bent that appealed to social elites; they called for autonomous healing through self-discipline, not the indulgent submissiveness of the rest cure. In this way, mind cure answered the urban gentry's desire to find an uplifting and private method of maintaining self-control and achieving psychic renewal. Through the cultivation of quiet, bodily rest, and isolation from the turmoil of modern society, sufferers could efficiently husband their psychic energies, gain control of their emotions, and assuage the stresses that led to neurasthenia. It should be noted, however, that mind cure's ideal of repose was merely a means of accommodation. It proposed not to cure society of its nervousness by backing away from "progress," but rather to help offset the deleterious effects of involvements in the business world and other challenging mental arenas. Achieved through a mind-cure regimen, repose was thus a morally upstanding and non-threatening panacea for nervousness that was readily accepted by the cultural elite.

Dewing made mind cure's ideal of physical and emotional balance central to his work. As the critic Royal Cortissoz noted, "There is never a plangent element in [Dewing's work]; . . . For startling emphasis he has no predilection. It would obscure the clarity, dislocate the steadiness of his serene vision."[30] Another critic observed the effortless bodily equilibrium demonstrated by Dewing's women, such as those in *Lady in White* and *Young Girl Seated*:

> When his women lean back in a chair you feel the just weight of the body, the exact amount that the arm is supporting the head, the exact amount the arm is being supported by the chair. You feel acutely, for he gives you exactly, the good thrusts and balances that are the structure of these women's repose.[31]

Stating that Dewing's women "are not the restless women of today," Catherine Beach Ely also observed that Dewing "perfectly understands the structure of the figure, its beautiful balance in repose." She therefore concluded that his women are "never eager nor anxious, their nerves not toiling and spinning, but in equilibrium."[32] The language and tone of these critics

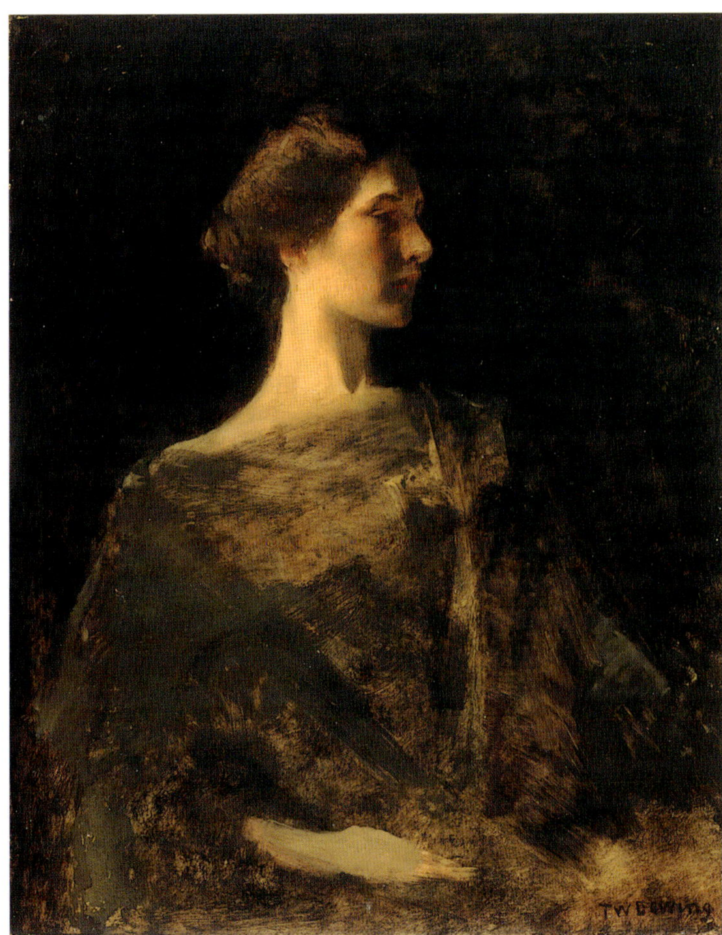

FIG. 15 Thomas Wilmer Dewing, *Alma*, c. 1895–1900. Oil on canvas, 20 × 15⅝ in. Smithsonian American Art Museum. Gift of John Gellatly.

on this point echo mind cure's pronouncements on repose almost verbatim; like Annie Payson Call and other mind-curists, Dewing subscribed to the ideals of rest and repose to ameliorate the stress of modern life.

The quiet atmosphere and evocation of physical and mental repose so typical of works such as *Lady in White*, *Young Girl Seated*, and *Alma* (fig. 15) established that Dewing's women were in complete control of their emotions—even to the extent that they had canceled their emotions altogether. Cortissoz asserted that "there is no drama in Dewing's *oeuvre*. There is no pathos, there is no sentiment, there is hardly any human interest at all. . . . Dewing's people have no emotions."[33] And Charles Caffin perceived that these women were "wrapt in a consciousness of self so complete that the consciousness is lost in a *dolce far*

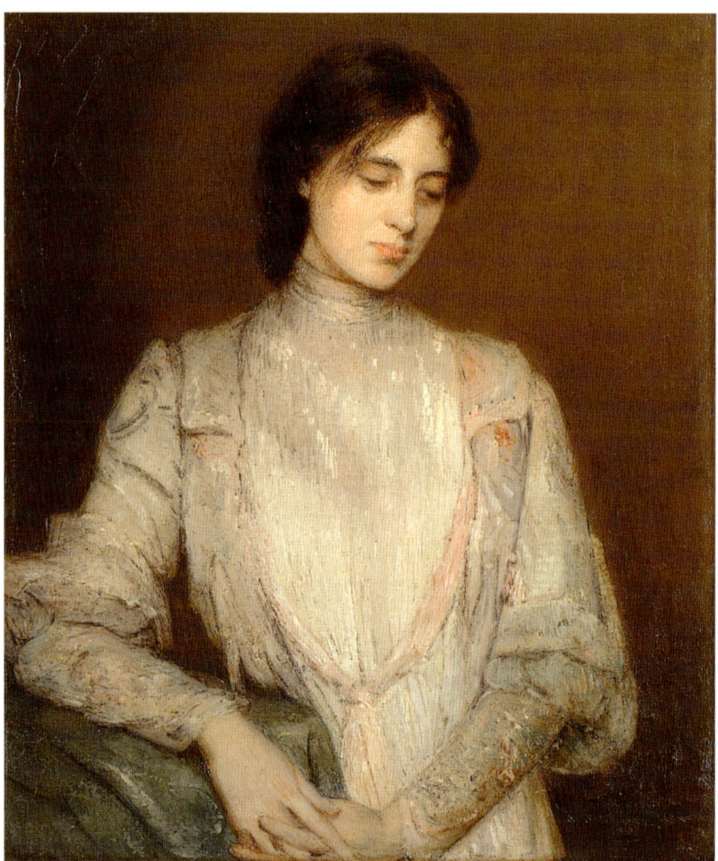

FIG. 16 Julian Alden Weir, *A Gentlewoman*, 1906.
Oil on canvas, 30 × 25 in. Smithsonian American
Art Museum. Gift of William T. Evans. 1909.7.72.

niente of feelingless existence."[34] Dewing's women were not subject to the Sturm und Drang of modern life but rather were insulated from nervousness by an idealized realm of nirvanic self-extinction.

One of the most common remarks voiced about Dewing's women concerned their high intelligence; Dewing was even known for selecting his models based on their "intellectual refinement."[35] From their calm, quiet, and relaxed composure and emotionless countenance, it was implicit that Dewing's women were free to use their minds to their fullest powers. Caffin believed that "Dewing's pictures create a feeling of extraordinary concentration" and that Dewing's women are of "a type in which the habit of intellectual control has clarified, but not effaced, the essential passionateness" of "intellectual emancipation."[36] Again we are reminded of Call's promise of the power that comes from the ability to "erase all previous impressions."

In addition to Dewing, many other American artists co-opted the mind-cure ideal of right thinking and self-control in constructing the Woman at Home. Julian Alden Weir's austere *A Gentlewoman* (fig. 16), typical of his studio paintings,[37] casts her weary gaze downward as she rests her arm languidly on a support at the left. The quiet mood and air of stillness are reinforced by the soft, glittering colors of her dress and the dark background against which she stands. The title of the work indicates this woman is of good breeding and is to be accorded appropriate respect; she upholds her station and does not saddle the family with her nervous worries. For although this woman is marked superficially by signs of nervousness, Weir gives her strength by presenting her upright—she leans gently but does not teeter—and renders her figure in convincing three-dimensional form. Instead of falling into morbid introspection, Weir's gentlewoman, praised for her "mixture of sturdiness and charm,"[38] pauses in a moment of productive thought.

Artists added to the Woman at Home's restorative potential by engaging the therapeutic discourse of interior decoration. The construction of a comfortable and harmoniously decorated interior environment where repose could be fostered was a favored prescription for releasing stress and avoiding nervousness.[39] Paintings such as Walter Launt Palmer's *De Forest Interior* (fig. 17) attest to the shared interests of painters and decorators. Commissioned by Henry F. de Forest, Palmer presumably portrays Mrs. de Forest at rest in her New York City home, the interior of which was designed by the de Forests' son, the noted decorator and Palmer's close friend, Lockwood de Forest.[40] The dark tones and orderly patterns of the Turkish-inspired decorative motifs, recreated painstakingly on the canvas by Palmer, create an atmosphere of tranquility and rest that is echoed in the comfortably relaxed figure of the seated woman. The scale of this splendid room, which dwarfs the reposing figure, alludes to the vastness of the restorative energies available to her. Believing that

FIG. 17 [*facing*] Walter Launt Palmer, *De Forest Interior*, 1878.
Oil on canvas, 24⅛ × 18 in. Smithsonian American Art
Museum. Museum Purchase 1982.46.

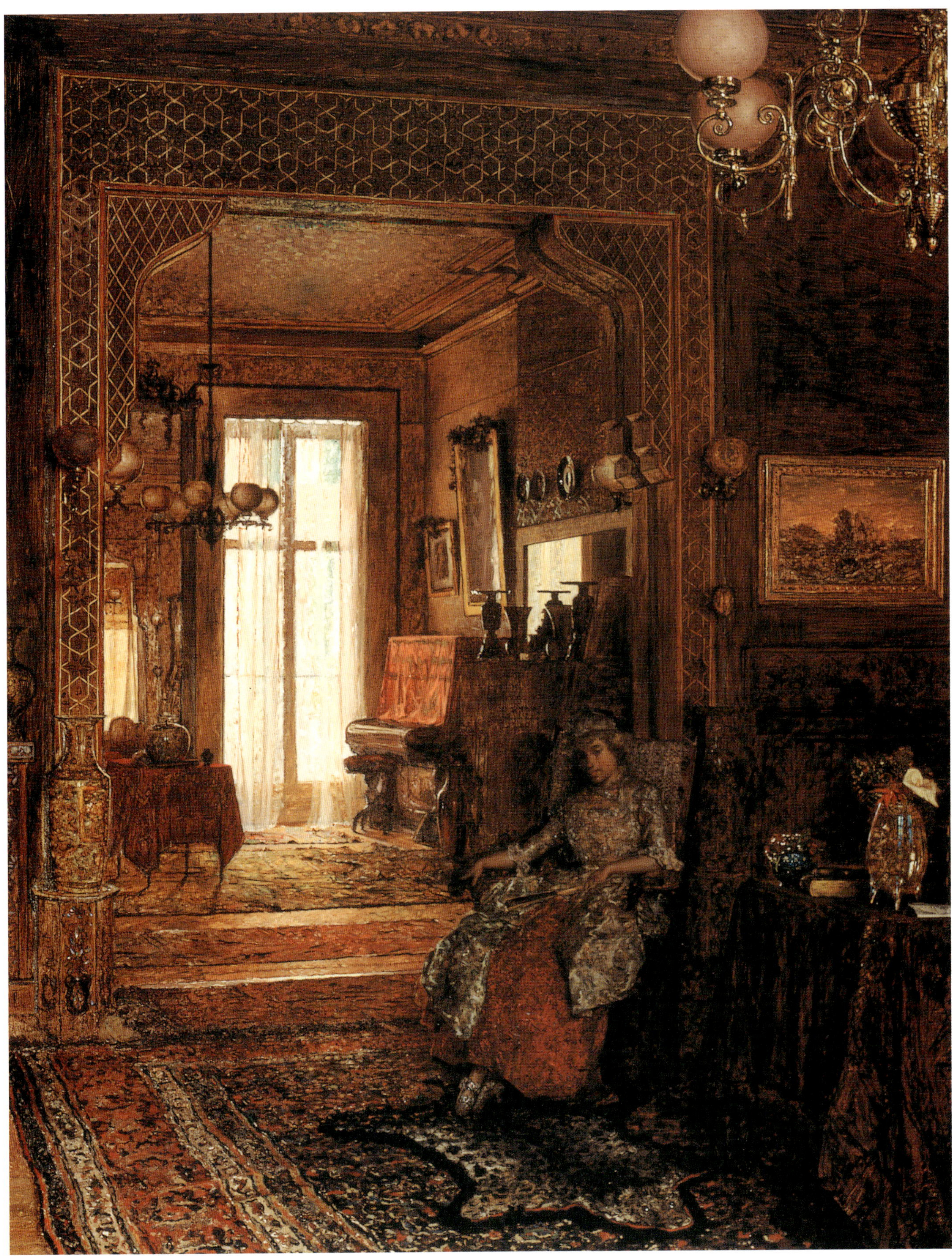

paintings "should not inspire headaches but participate in the restful ambiance of the domestic environment,"[41] artists such as Palmer shared with their decorator compatriots an allied concern for gentle rhythms, tonal harmonies, and the creation of an aesthetic space for physical and mental repose. Aiming to collapse the divide between art and life, artists and decorators like Palmer and de Forest sought "to enrich a quotidian existence by submitting consciousness to the stylization and ritualization of art; to induce a state of inward repose through outer material beauty."[42] Similarly, the spare settings of such works as Dewing's *Lady in White*, which portrays a woman in a minimally furnished interior, express a simplified notion of taste and refinement. This aesthetic choice implies restraint, a calm ordering of the interior that protects its occupants from external forces.[43] The emptiness of the space around Dewing's woman is analogous to the mind freed from nervous anxieties. Thus insulated, this ambient space represents a safe haven where the woman's anxieties dissipate in an atmosphere of abundant, soothing, restorative energy.

The Woman at Home occupies the intersection of these therapeutic ideals: the tastefully arranged and harmoniously decorated domestic interior, its occupant in repose, recapitulates the painting's message of healthful rest emblemized by the reclining woman whose figure is a study in equipoise. Paintings of the Woman at Home function therapeutically by suggesting transport to an orderly inner sanctum far removed from the outer world, which is riven by contradictory forces. Returning once again to Dewing's *Lady in White*, we can see how this formula was realized by one of the leading practitioners of the Woman at Home genre. With her body relaxed and her emotions in check, the woman's self-control overcomes her inclinations toward nervousness. Harmony of design is equated with harmony of mind; tonal gradations of soothing color—explicitly evoking the oceanic realm of spiritual energy promised by mind cure—ameliorate the hostile energies of modern society. The message is positive: the *Lady in White* transcends anxieties arising from the stress of modern life, and she offers an instructional model for the viewer in insulating himself from his own neurasthenic inclinations.

Another artist who made the Woman at Home a major component of his oeuvre was John White Alexander. Alexander was the primary American exponent of a decorative, art nouveau style of figure painting joined with a tonalist palette derived from Whistler. He was also a confirmed neurasthenic who nonetheless worked tirelessly as both an artist and a leader in art organizations, including serving as the president of the National Academy of Design.[44] Alexander's views on art were colored by his own nervous sensitivity; he once asserted "that one's conception of beauty depends largely upon one's mood, the condition of one's nerves, [and] one's circulation and digestion."[45] Critics projected the artist's own nervousness onto his works, valorizing his "singularly flexible and sensitive" "nervous temperament" as the source of his aesthetic refinement.[46] Following Whistler's example, Alexander labored to produce an art of repose through an analogy with music, emphasizing gentle contours and subtle rhythms, and rendered his paintings in an array of muted colors. In his appropriately titled *Repose* (fig. 18), Alexander emphasizes the graceful curves of the recumbent woman, who looks back toward the picture plane with an expression of dolorous indifference. While ostensibly tired and in need of rest, this woman has not a care in the world as she indulges in an afternoon of playful reverie. The flowing lines of her figure and the curves of the couch animate the composition and imbue it with a rhythmic energy, as if to demonstrate the restorative potential of rest and relaxation.

Alexander extended these ideas to his work in portraiture. In *Portrait of Miss Dorothy Roosevelt (Mrs. Langdon Geer)* he portrays his sitter in a relaxed posture and seated in a comfortable chair, her weary eyes cast downward in a moment of contemplation (see frontispiece). Alexander follows the therapeutic template for the typical Woman at Home painting. His application of paint is thin and his brushstroke smooth and freely applied, his use of color warm and composed of closely allied hues. The interior space is spare, the atmosphere relaxed. Alexander adds to the air of tranquility by

FIG. 18 [*facing*] John White Alexander, *Repose*, 1895. Oil on canvas, 52¼ × 63⅝ in. The Metropolitan Museum of Art, Anonymous Gift, 1980 (1980.244).

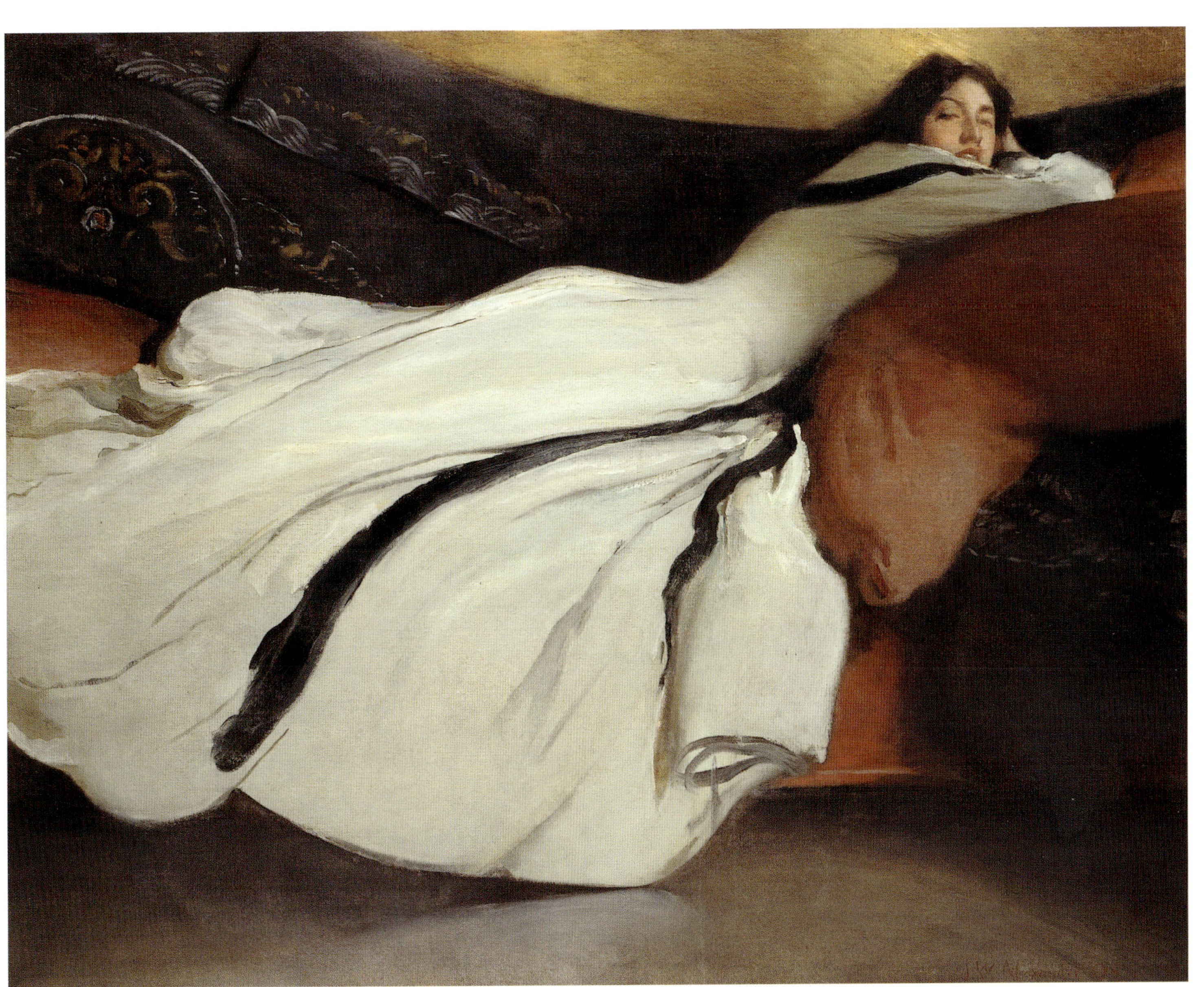

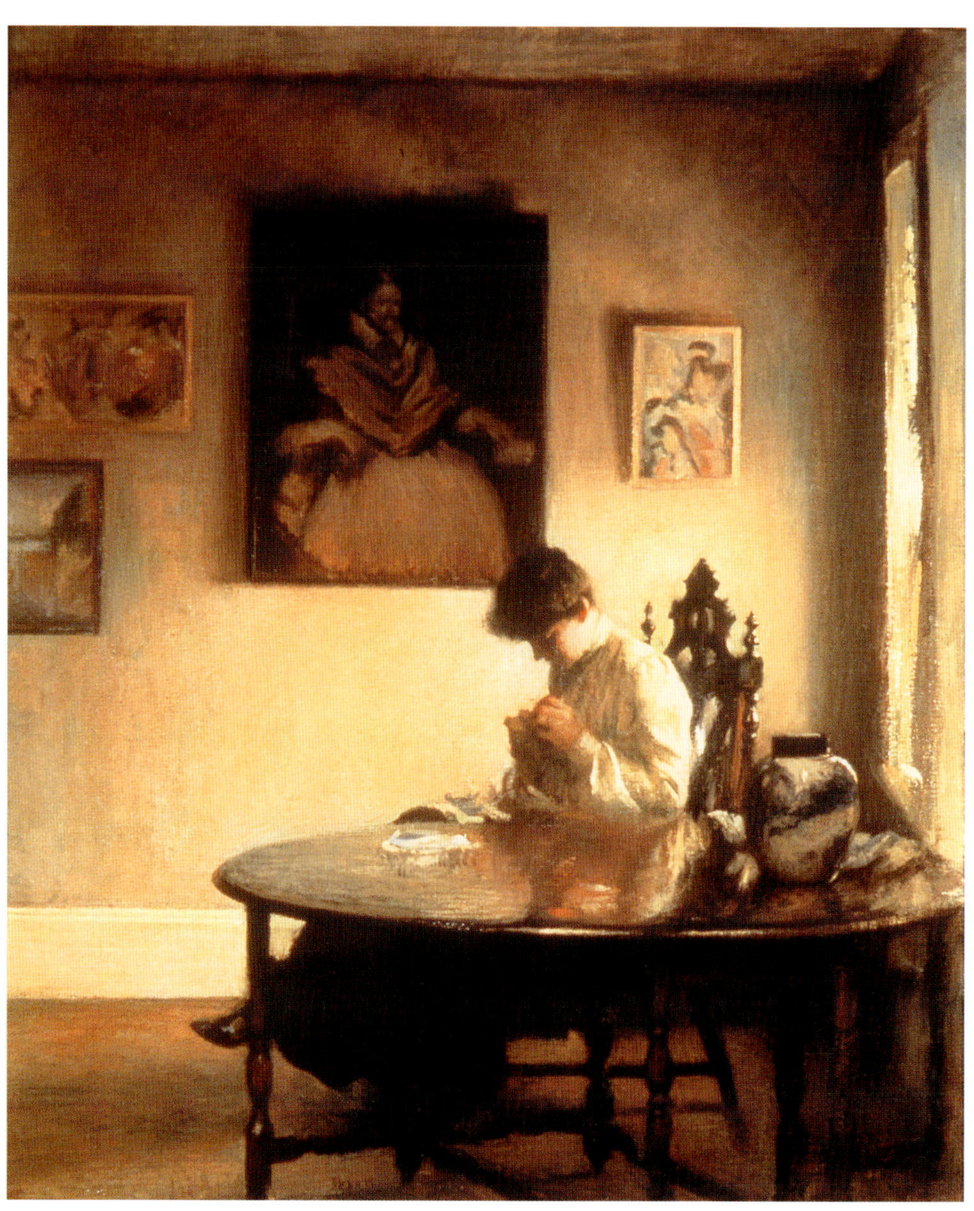

echoing Miss Roosevelt's attitude of repose in the slumbering presence of the large setter dog, who lies listlessly on the floor. While her weary appearance hints at nervous strain (and thus her genteel refinement), Miss Roosevelt's thoughts are far away as she is absorbed by the warm light that bathes the spare interior.

The Woman at Home motif was developed enthusiastically by the leader of the Boston School, Edmund Tarbell. After beginning his professional career in the 1890s as a plein air painter in the impressionist mode, by the early 1900s Tarbell reformulated his work under the influence of the seventeenth-century Dutch masters, especially Pieter de Hooch and Johannes Vermeer.[47] The revival of interest in Vermeer in this period, particularly among painters of the Boston School— for example, Frank Weston Benson, Joseph DeCamp, William MacGregor Paxton, and Philip Leslie Hale— has been related to the "psychological need for repose" of the Gilded Age.[48] The girl in Tarbell's famous *Girl Crocheting* (fig. 19) follows Vermeer's prototype. Tarbell's girl crochets meditatively by the soft window light, her mind lost in the relaxing, aesthetic joy of craft. This idealized scene of domestic tranquility evokes the quiet and calm cherished by Tarbell's world-weary Boston patrons—exemplary New England "brain workers" who were principally "collectors whose wealth was based in a mercantile economy."[49]

At the height of the Gilded Age, the Woman at Home achieved widespread popularity among artists and collectors. Preoccupied with neurasthenia, America's elite population sought private and morally upstanding methods of relaxation to transport their worried consciences far from the stresses of modern society. Situated amidst the discourses of mind cure and interior decoration, paintings of the Woman at Home by Dewing, Weir, Alexander, and others depicted quiet, intimate spaces of rest and relaxation. Sounding a positive note in an era of discord, these artists presented women in the process of overcoming neurasthenia through self-control, creating paintings

FIG. 19 [*facing*] Edmund Tarbell, *Girl Crocheting*, 1904. Oil on canvas, 30 × 24 in. Canajoharie Library and Art Gallery, Canajoharie, New York.

that served as visual cues to help induce repose and replenish the weary soul.

The Woman at Home genre declined in popularity in the early years of the twentieth century. A multitude of factors helped usher out the Woman at Home from her position of prominence, but among the most important of them was the rise of an anti-genteel bias in American culture that increasingly identified energy, dynamism, and vitality as quintessentially American attributes to the detriment of "refinement" and "taste." Action, not rest, became the preferred tonic for weary nerves. The Woman at Home, symbolic of escapist repose, began to lose her potency as a counteragent to nervousness. Furthermore, women's increasing visibility in the workplace could no longer be denied. This diminished their potential as symbols of relaxation, and paintings of genteel ladies resting came to be seen as anachronistic.[50] They were soon supplanted by the idealized images of the Gibson Girl, a dynamic female archetype who celebrated her sexuality and freedom of action while retaining her genteel charm. Finally, by the 1920s neurasthenia itself fell out of favor in the medical establishment, as new treatments for mental illness, especially Freudian psychoanalysis, began to attribute neuroses to subconscious, and not physical, forces. Psychoanalysis offered salvation from neuroses through the patient's self-discovery, quite the opposite of mind cure's program of self-extinction.[51] The Woman at Home, in this emerging paradigm of mental health, lost her potency as a symbol of emotional release and no longer had the power to heal injured nerves.

Notes

This essay would not have been possible without the help of Claire Perry and Wanda Corn, who each gave great advice and insight during its development.

1. The general trend in scholarship on paintings of women in interior settings, and the construction of ideal beauty that the paintings promoted, has been to highlight the paintings' negative, "antifeminist" attributes: they deny the new, socially liberal roles for women that were enabled through advances in women's suffrage; they reinforce conservative "separate-sphere" ideology by pictorially representing women trapped in domestic spaces; and by picturing women "doing nothing" they objectify women's

bodies as mere decorative elements within the composition. Each of these readings does much to explain why the woman-in-interior motif had such powerful cultural significance in this period. By reinforcing woman's proscribed role in fostering a harmonious domestic environment and denying her the freedoms of the "New Woman," these paintings downplayed challenges to male hegemony over the established social order. The most influential source to articulate these ideas is Bernice Kramer Leader, "Antifeminism in the Paintings of the Boston School," *Arts Magazine* 56 (January 1982): 112–19. Other important sources on women in interiors are Martha Banta, *Imaging American Women: Idea and Ideals in Cultural History* (New York: Columbia University Press, 1987), especially 339–74; Bailey Van Hook, *Angels of Art: Women and Art in American Society, 1876–1914* (University Park: The Pennsylvania State University Press, 1996); Beverly Gordon, "Woman's Domestic Body: The Conceptual Conflation of Women and Interiors in the Industrial Age," *Winterthur Portfolio* 30, no. 1 (Spring 1995): 281–99; Julie Anne Springer, "Art and the Feminine Muse: Women in Interiors by John White Alexander," *Woman's Art Journal* 6, no. 2 (Fall 1985/Winter 1986): 1–8; and Celia Betsky, "In the Artist's Studio," *Portfolio* 4, no. 1 (January/February 1982): 32–39. Another article that addresses the tendency to treat women as decorative objects is Annette Stott, "Floral Femininity: A Pictorial Definition," *American Art* 6, no. 2 (Spring 1992): 37–60. Carroll Smith-Rosenberg, "The New Woman as Androgyne: Social Disorder and Gender Crisis, 1870–1936," in *Disorderly Conduct: Visions of Gender in Victorian America* (New York: Alfred A. Knopf, 1985), 245–96, discusses the social implications of many of the new roles women performed in this period.

2. Here I follow the lead of Martha Banta, who has proposed more positive readings of paintings of women in interiors. She asserts that "it was ill considered at the time and . . . it still is to assume that the use of conventions which portray women in outward attitudes reflective of inward stillness are gross evidence of the moral turpitude of an entire culture," 365.

3. On Gilded Age cultural changes, see Alan Trachtenberg, *The Incorporation of America: Culture & Society in the Gilded Age* (New York: Hill and Wang, 1982), esp. 3–10, and T. J. Jackson Lears, *No Place of Grace: Antimodernism and the Transformation of American Culture, 1880–1920* (New York: Pantheon Books, 1981), 4–11.

4. George M. Beard, *American Nervousness: Its Causes and Consequences* (New York: G. P. Putnam's Sons, 1881).

5. Tom Lutz, *American Nervousness, 1903: An Anecdotal History* (Ithaca, NY: Cornell University Press, 1991), esp. 3–7. On gendered readings of neurasthenia, see Elaine Showalter, *The Female Malady: Women, Madness, and English Culture, 1830–1980* (New York: Pantheon Books, 1985), 135; Ann Douglas Wood, "'The Fashionable Diseases': Women's Complaints and Their Treatment in Nineteenth-Century America," in *Clio's Conscious-*

ness Raised: New Perspectives on the History of Women, ed. Mary S. Hartman and Lois Banner (New York: Harper Collins Books, 1974), 2; and Carol Bauer and Lawrence Ritt, "'The Little Health of Ladies': An Anatomy of Female Invalidism in the Nineteenth Century," *Journal of the American Medical Women's Association* 36 (1981): 300–306.

6. Dewing has drawn significant attention from scholars in recent years. Susan A. Hobbs's *The Art of Thomas Wilmer Dewing: Beauty Reconfigured*, exh. cat. (Washington, D.C.: The Smithsonian Institution Press, in association with The Brooklyn Museum, 1996) is the definitive biography. Kathleen Pyne has written extensively on Dewing and Spencerian evolution, particularly in the chapter "Aesthetic Strategies in the Age of Pain" in her *Art and the Higher Life: Painting and Evolutionary Thought in Late Nineteenth-Century America* (Austin: University of Texas Press, 1996), 135–219.

7. On sources, see Judith Elizabeth Lyczko, "Thomas Wilmer Dewing's Sources: Women in Interiors," *Arts Magazine* 54, no. 3 (September 1979): 152–57.

8. Pyne has established Dewing's connection to the therapeutic worldview of the period; see especially 158–63.

9. Catherine Beach Ely, "Thomas W. Dewing," *Art in America and Elsewhere* 10 (August 1922): 225.

10. On Freer and nervousness, see Lears, 190, and Pyne, 168. On Freer and release from tension, see Hobbs, 24.

11. There have been many treatments of the rest cure; see especially Ellen L. Bassuk, "The Rest Cure: Repetition or Resolution of Victorian Women's Conflicts?" in *The Female Body in Western Culture*, ed. Susan Rubin Suleiman (Cambridge, MA: Harvard University Press, 1986), 139–51.

12. Kathleen Spies argues persuasively for a neurasthenic reading of the portraits of Thomas Eakins in her essay in this catalogue (37–51).

13. On negative perception of female neurasthenia, see George Frederick Drinka, *The Birth of Neurosis: Myth, Malady and the Victorians* (New York: Simon & Schuster, 1984), 202–9.

14. See, for example, Ruth McEnery Stuart, *The Cocoon: A Rest-Cure Comedy* (New York: Hearst's International Library Co., 1915); Augustus Hoppin, *A Fashionable Sufferer; or, Chapters from Life's Comedy* (New York: Houghton, Mifflin and Company, 1883); Gertrude E. Jennings, "A Rest Cure," in *Four One-Act Plays* (New York: Samuel French, 1914); and William B. Maxwell, *The Rest Cure, a Novel* (New York: Appleton, 1910).

15. On invalidism in America, see Erika Ingelin Rozinek, "'We All Take Our Turn': Invalidism in American Culture, 1850–1910," master's thesis (Newark: University of Delaware, 2003).

16. Christian Brinton, *Modern Artists* (New York: Baker and Taylor, 1908), 112.

17. Sarah Burns, *Inventing the Modern Artist: Art and Culture in the Gilded Age* (New Haven: Yale University Press, 1996), 135.

18. On the experience of art as a transforming moment, see Pyne, 177.

19. Sarah Burns, "Revitalizing the 'Painted Out' North: Winslow Homer, Manly Health, and New England Regionalism in Turn-of-the-Century America," *American Art* 9, no. 2 (Summer 1995): 21–38.

20. Van Hook, 169, and Pyne, 183.

21. On art and mind cure, see Pyne, 155–57, and Burns, 139–40. The best sources on mind cure in general are Gail Thain Parker, *Mind Cure in New England: From the Civil War to World War I* (Hanover, NH: University Press of New England, 1973), and Donald Meyer, *The Positive Thinkers: Popular Religious Psychology from Mary Baker Eddy to Norman Vincent Peale and Ronald Reagan* (Middletown, CT: Wesleyan University Press, 1988).

22. S. Weir Mitchell, *Wear and Tear, or Hints for the Over-worked* (Philadelphia: J. B. Lippincott & Co., 1871). "The gospel of work must make way for the gospel of rest," Beard, 313.

23. William James, *The Varieties of Religious Experience* (Cambridge, MA: Harvard University Press, 1985), 83.

24. Barbara Sicherman, "The Paradox of Prudence: Mental Health in the Gilded Age," *The Journal of American History* 62, no. 4 (March 1976): 894; and Bassuk, 143.

25. William S. Sadler, *Worry and Nervousness: The Science of Self-Mastery* (Chicago: A. C. McClurg & Co., 1914), 329.

26. Annie Payson Call, *Power Through Repose* (Boston: Roberts Brothers, 1891). For a discussion of Call and mind cure, see Parker, 82–86.

27. Call, 34.

28. Ibid., 139.

29. J. W. Courtney, "Hygiene of the Brain and Nervous System," in *A Manual of Personal Hygiene: Proper Living Upon a Physiological Basis*, ed. Walter L. Pyle (Philadelphia: W. B. Saunders, 1901), 300.

30. Royal Cortissoz, "An American Artist Canonized in the Freer Gallery," *Scribner's Magazine* 77, no. 5 (November 1923): 545–46.

31. Ezra Tharp, "T. W. Dewing," *Art and Progress* 5, no. 5 (March 1914): 156.

32. Ely, 225, 226.

33. Cortissoz, 544.

34. Charles H. Caffin, "Some American Portrait Painters," *The Critic* 44, no. 1 (January 1904): 36.

35. Charles H. Caffin, "The Art of Thomas W. Dewing," *Harper's Monthly Magazine* 116, no. 495 (April 1908): 722.

36. Ibid., 723–24.

37. Doreen Bolder Burke, *J. Alden Weir: An American Impressionist* (Newark: University of Delaware Press, 1983), 243.

38. Charles De Kay, "The World of Art and Artists," *New York Times*, January 21, 1906, 8.

39. On the development of a therapeutic interior in response to neurasthenia, see Keith Bresnahan, "Neurasthenic Subjects and the Bourgeois Interior," *Space & Culture* 6, no. 2 (May 2003): 169–77; Joyce Henri Robinson, "'Hi honey, I'm home': Weary (Neurasthenic) Businessmen and the Formulation of a Serenely Modern Aesthetic," in *Not at Home: The Suppression of Domesticity in Modern Art and Architecture*, ed. Christopher Reed (London: Thames & Hudson, 1996), 98–112; and Burns, 142–43. In at least one case interior decorations were used for the actual medical treatment of neurasthenia; see *Art Collector* 9, no. 3 (December 1, 1898): 41–42.

40. Teresa A. Carbone, *At Home with Art: Paintings in American Interiors, 1780–1920*, exh. cat. (New York: Katonah Museum of Art, 1995), 32. Neither Palmer nor Lockwood de Forest has received much scholarly attention. The only comprehensive treatment of Palmer's life and works is Maybelle Mann, *Walter Launt Palmer: Poetic Reality* (Exton, PA: Schiffer Pub. Ltd., 1984), while Anne Suydam Lewis's slender *Lockwood de Forest: Painter, Importer, Decorator*, exh. cat. (Huntington, NY: Heckscher Museum, 1976), remains the definitive monograph on the artist.

41. Robinson, 103.

42. Pyne, 165.

43. Van Hook, 168.

44. The most comprehensive treatment of Alexander's life and career is Sarah J. Moore, *John White Alexander and the Construction of National Identity: Cosmopolitan American Art, 1880–1915* (Newark: University of Delaware Press, 2003). For Alexander's own nervousness, see Springer, 3.

45. "Need Good Digestion to Appreciate Beauty," *New York Evening Mail*, December 10, 1910, 5.

46. Christian Brinton, "The Art of John W. Alexander," *Munsey's Magazine* 39, no. 6 (September 1908): 753. On the phenomenon of reading Alexander's work in light of his nervousness, see Springer, 3.

47. Erica E. Hirshler, "'Good and Beautiful Work': Edmund C. Tarbell and the Arts and Crafts Movement," in *Impressionism Transformed: The Paintings of Edmund C. Tarbell*, exhib. cat., ed. Susan Strickler (Manchester, NH: The Currier Museum of Art, 2001), 86.

48. Springer, 3.

49. Hirshler, 86.

50. Van Hook, 209–13.

51. Francis G. Gosling, *Before Freud: Neurasthenia and the American Medical Community, 1870–1910* (Urbana: University of Illinois Press, 1987), 164–72.

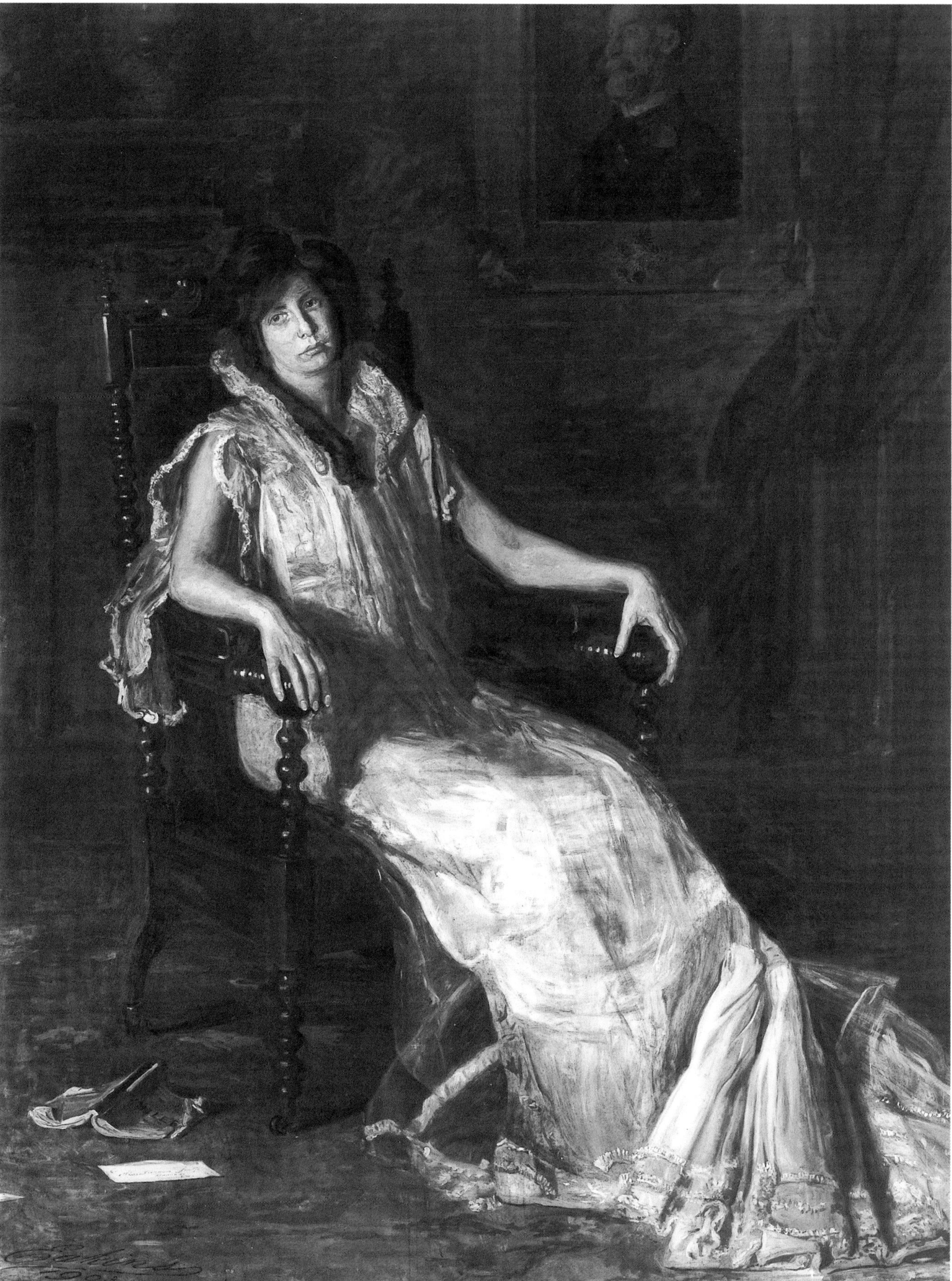

KATHLEEN SPIES

FIGURING THE NEURASTHENIC

THOMAS EAKINS, NERVOUS ILLNESS, AND GENDER IN VICTORIAN AMERICA

he melancholy tone and signs of weariness in the portraits of Philadelphia painter Thomas Eakins (1844–1916) have long been acknowledged. Indeed, the slouched posture, teary eyes, and tilted head of Suzanne Santje in *The Actress* (fig. 20) convey a sense of exhaustion and depression, as do the downcast gaze, drawn features, and emaciated figure of *Frank Hamilton Cushing* (fig. 21). However, these indications of physical, mental, and/or emotional fatigue have given rise to widely divergent readings. Whereas Santje's portrait has been thought to represent "the mysterious beauty … of sadness"[1] and to show the actress "in a state of near collapse," Cushing's portrait has been seen as a "tribute to [Cushing's] daring and contributions to social science,"[2] revealing "the moral force of intellect."[3] What did Eakins bring to these paintings that would encourage such varied reactions?

While recent Eakins scholarship attends to gender issues, it often fails to sufficiently connect these issues with the pervasive weariness shown in the portraits and, additionally, to treat this weariness within the context of period thoughts on chronic exhaustion and fatigue, most predominantly encompassed by the nervous illness that was known as "neurasthenia." It is my

contention that an exploration of Eakins's portraits of men and women at this intersection of gender and illness will enable us to understand better the divergent responses to the artist's works, as well as the subtle and elusive coding of the paintings themselves. As society perceived female and male neurasthenics in dramatically different ways, Eakins's portraits both reflected and contributed to these perceptions.[4] Malleable in definition, neurasthenia functioned for the artist and his culture as a means of exaggerating and encompassing already-present gender myths, providing explanations for the otherwise inexplicable. It unified seemingly irreconcilable contradictions and served to control tensions both in the artist's personal life and in the wider culture of nineteenth-century America.

Also known as "nervous exhaustion" or simply as "nervousness," neurasthenia referred to a weakness of the nerves and a depletion of energy or "nerve force" that resulted in tiredness or depression. For roughly forty years following the coining of the term in 1869 by physician George Beard—notably the time span of Eakins's

FIG. 20 [*facing*] Thomas Eakins, *The Actress*, 1903. Oil on canvas, 80 × 60 in. Philadelphia Museum of Art. Given by Mrs. Thomas Eakins and Miss Mary Adeline Williams.

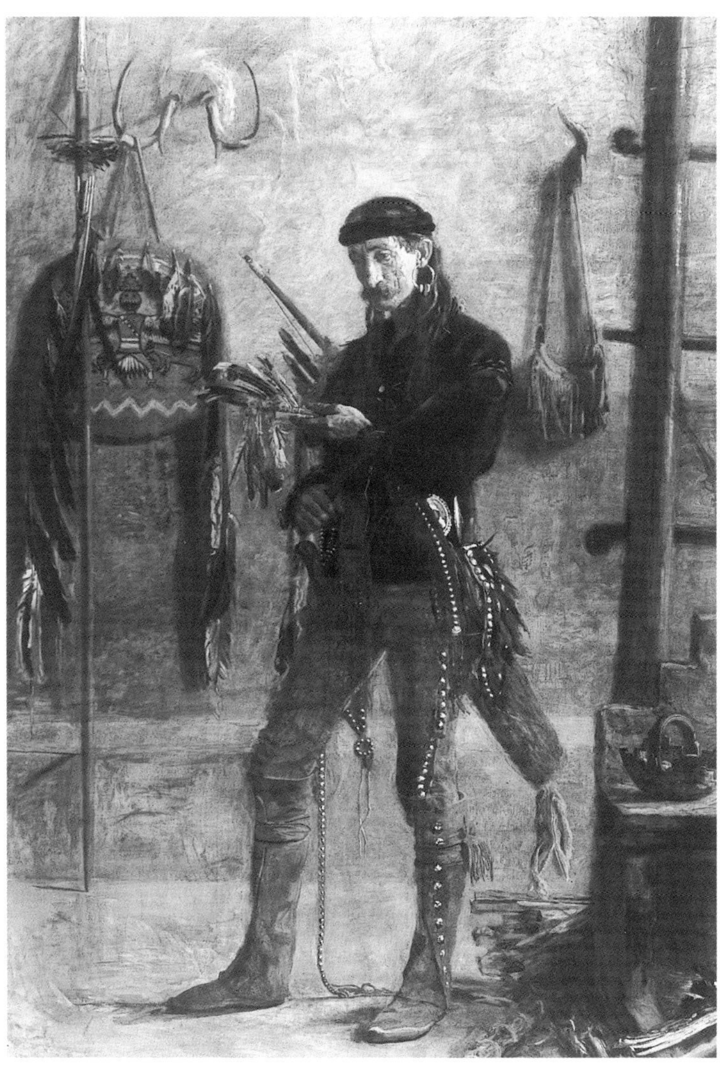

FIG. 21 Thomas Eakins, *Frank Hamilton Cushing*, 1895.
Oil on canvas, 90 × 60 in. Courtesy of the
Gilcrease Museum, Tulsa, Oklahoma.

activity—neurasthenia spread throughout America's
medical and popular culture to almost epidemic proportions. Three hundred and thirty-two articles were
published on nervousness in medical journals alone.
A household word at the time,[5] neurasthenia confronted Victorians in advice books and columns of
popular magazines, in novels by Edith Wharton and
Theodore Dreiser, and in advertisements, such as that
for Winchester's Specific Pill, which claimed to cure
"Nervousness: Exhausted or Debilitated Nerve Force."
Eakins himself had a bout with the illness in 1886 and
knew numerous others who suffered from the sickness;
he was even friends with doctors who specialized in its

treatment. By the turn of the twentieth century neurasthenic language was so pervasive that it infiltrated the
discourses of economics, religion, politics, and industry,
producing terms such as "nervous bankruptcy."[6]

Definitions of the illness remained vague, however,
and its frequency, symptoms, causes, and cures all varied greatly according to the patient. As neurasthenia
was primarily considered an affliction of the white middle and upper classes, these differences were typically
based on gender rather than on race or class. Like
numerous physicians of his time, Eakins typed his
female sitters as ill or on the brink of illness while
showing the male neurasthenic as an anomaly of his
sex. According to contemporaries, a woman was susceptible because she had a highly emotional nature
and disease-prone sex organs that dictated her entire
being. Although it is difficult to recover the realities of
nineteenth-century women's health, the female invalid was a standard feature in American culture by the
mid-1800s.[7]

Such a climate resulted in statements such as that
by S. Weir Mitchell, a friend of Eakins and a prominent neurologist in the artist's hometown of Philadelphia, who claimed, "The man who does not know sick
women does not know women."[8] For Eakins, perhaps
typing his female sitters as neurasthenic functioned as
it did for the physicians—as a method to understand
that which seemed impossible to understand, as a
means of fitting problematic, mysterious, and confusing
women into a neatly defined and understandable, scientific category. Indeed, with the sparse and repetitive
format of *Addie* (c. 1900), *Miss Alice Kurtz* (fig. 22), *Clara*
(c. 1900), *Lucy Lewis* (1896), *Maud Cook* (1895), and
numerous others, these portraits appear similar to
pathological studies. Not only does the artist consistently pose his sitters with tilted heads, downcast or
sidelong gazes, and a three-quarter turn of the body,
but he also often employs a blank background and
a close-up bust format that further accentuates this
categorization. Unlike the majority of portraits of the
period, including those by John Singer Sargent, which
emphasized lush surfaces and material surroundings,
the scientific quality of these works instead places them
closer to Eakins's anatomical photographs and medical

paintings such as *The Agnew Clinic*, in which several male medical assistants probe a diseased female body (fig. 23).

Other details in Eakins's portraits of women further contribute to the paintings' resemblance to pathological studies and point more directly to the symptoms of female neurasthenia. Completed in the mid-1880s, *Portrait of a Lady with a Setter Dog* (fig. 24) is a portrait of the artist's wife, who, although said to be lively and energetic, is here shown with a dull expression, weary and teary-eyed, slouching under an emotional heaviness. The overall tone is dark, with the dramatic lighting calling attention to the wrinkles on her face and the bags under her eyes. Her dress is wrinkled and unkempt as well, adding to this sense of emotional disarray. Lines droop and slope downwards in a weighty manner that is emphasized by the heavy curtain behind the sitter. Throughout the production of this painting, Eakins made alterations to his wife's frame so that her shoulders would appear smaller, making her seem even more frail and vulnerable.[9] The most blatant sign of this weakness and weariness, however, lies at the very center of the painting, where the sitter's unusually large hand lies upward and open on her lap, impotent and useless. In all, the portrait seems to illustrate Mitchell's observation regarding the female neurasthenic: "everything wearies her—to sew, to write, to read, to walk."[10]

Eakins consistently repeated iconographic elements throughout his portraits of women. Almost without exception, all are shown in a state of complete inactivity with slouched, tired postures, heavy limbs, and tear-filled eyes. Along with wearily tilted heads and disheveled hair and clothes, these signs point to a state of depression, physical exhaustion, and a tendency to cry, the three most commonly noted symptoms of neurasthenia in both medical and popular literature. With dark colors, dramatic lighting, and downward sloping or jagged lines, the artist further intensified the general tone of melancholy and emotional trauma.

More specific indications of neurasthenia can be found in the carefully rendered details of the face. In *Mrs. Talcott Williams* (1891), for example, the sitter's red, mottled face, pout, and upturned eyebrows indicate teariness—a disturbed state that again is echoed by the

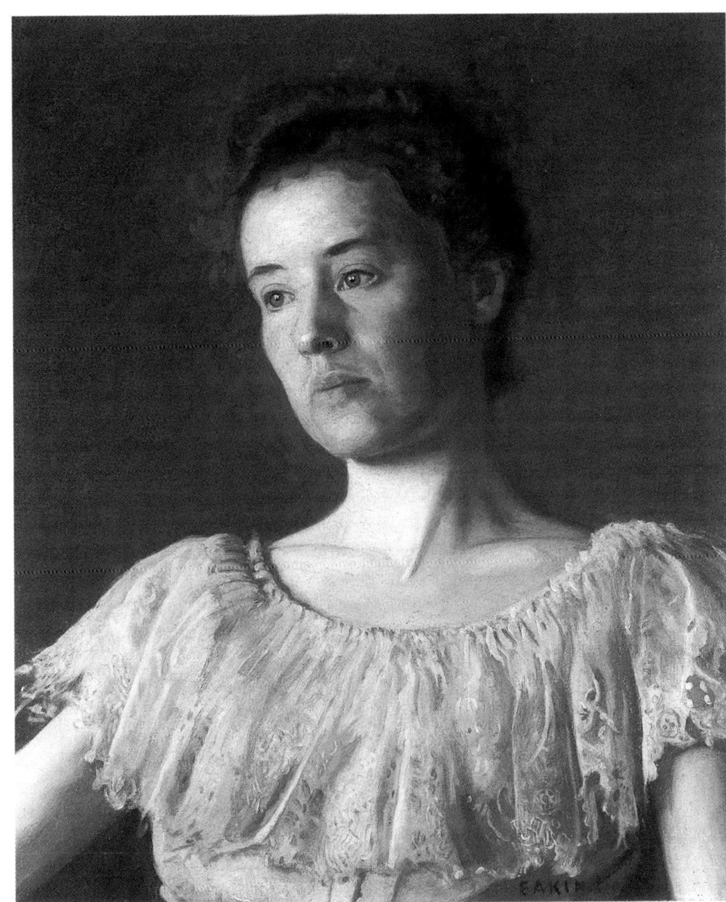

FIG. 22 Thomas Eakins, *Miss Alice Kurtz*, 1903. Oil on canvas, 23 × 19 in. Fogg Art Museum, Harvard University Art Museums. Gift in part of Mrs. John Whiteman (Alice Kurtz); Purchase in part with funds contributed by friends of John Coolidge, Director, 1948–1968.

wrinkles and crimped folds of her evening gown. In *Clara*, Eakins depicts the eyes as bloodshot and moist and gives a tenseness to the chin that signals an attempt to repress additional crying. All of these expressions are in contrast to the pensive gaze and crinkled brow of the male subject in *Henry O. Tanner* (1902). The women in *The Old Fashioned Dress* (fig. 25) and *Letitia Wilson Jordan* (1888), among others, are shown with a vacant look. As a symptom attributed to the neurasthenic, the vacant stare was originally thought to occur immediately before or after the hysterical fit, and it was later seen as a sign of the neurasthenic's unawareness of her surroundings.[11] Like rumpled clothes and tousled hair, the vacant stare came to be incorporated into the repertoire of iconography used to indicate mental illness in

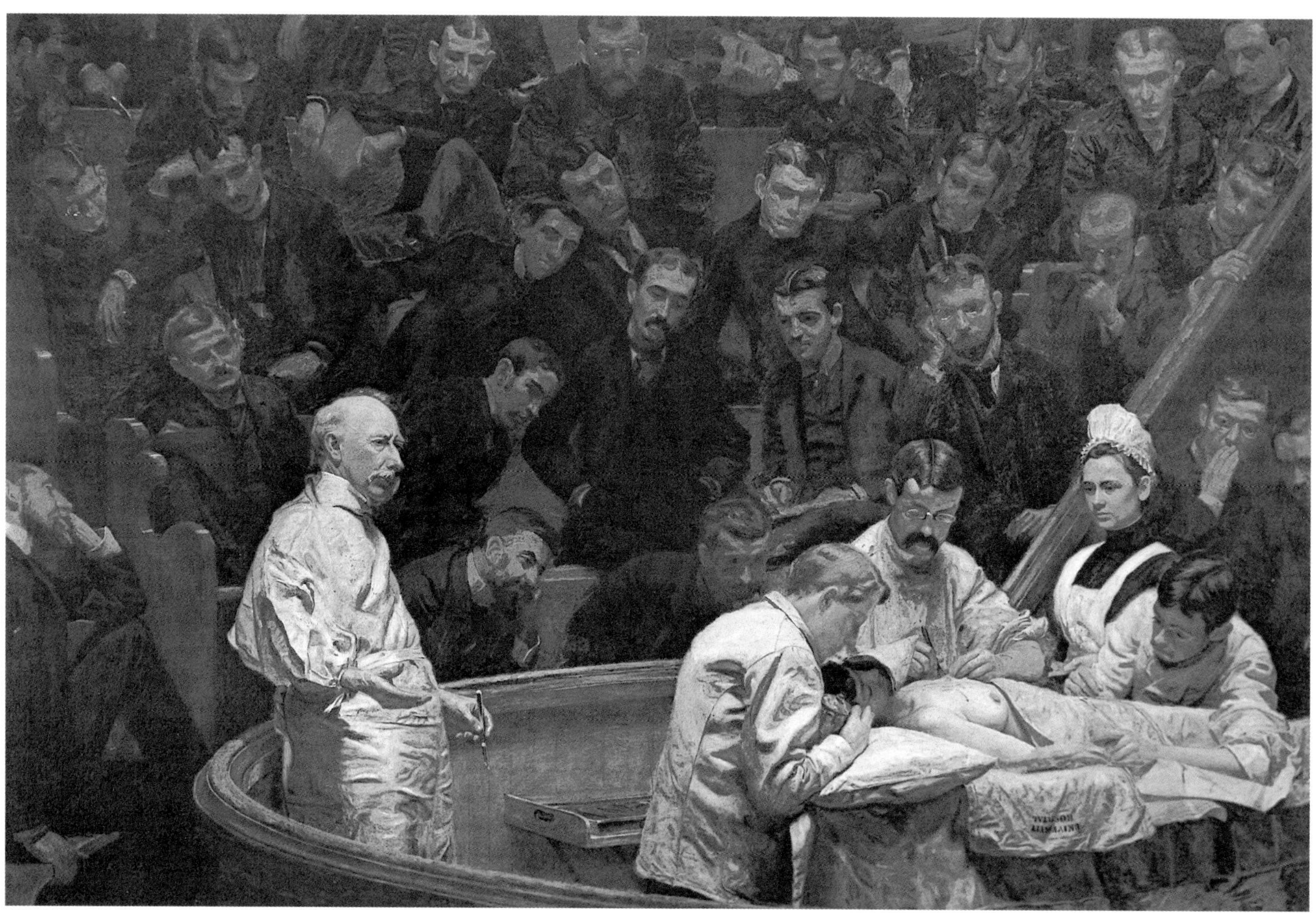

FIG. 23 Thomas Eakins, *The Agnew Clinic*, 1889. Oil on canvas,
84⅜ × 118⅛ in. University of Pennsylvania School of Medicine.

painting, and it gained the praise of critics when suc-
cessfully conveyed.[12] The precise detail given to Susan
Eakins's hand makes it seem stiff and heavy with
numbness, beyond weakness and perhaps even suggesting paralysis. In the portrait *Mary Hallock Greenewalt*
(1903), the hands again seem heavy and stiff, and the
neck appears extremely rigid as well.[13] Such muscular
difficulties, especially in the hands, were commonly
cited as symptoms and indications of nervousness.
In most cases, these "difficulties" referred to a general
weakness, but in some it meant the extremes of numbness, temporary paralysis, and catalepsy, a sudden hard-
ening or stiffness of the muscles.[14]

As he did his wife, Susan, Eakins usually painted
women in their upper middle age, adding years to the
younger sitters. Not only was menopause considered a

"disease-ridden time," but neurasthenics were sometimes noted to have aged and grayed prematurely due
to a high level of emotional stress.[15] A comparison of
Amelia Van Buren (1891) and a photo that shows the
sitter to be blond-haired and smooth-skinned reveals
Eakins's deliberate aging of Van Buren in the oil painting.[16] Eakins took the liberty of changing the appearance of other sitters as well. Helen Parker noted that
through subsequent stages of *The Old Fashioned Dress*,
Eakins painted her "really small and dainty nose more
and more bulbous," an exaggeration readily visible
when the painting is contrasted with a photograph

FIG. 24 [*facing*] Thomas Eakins, *Portrait of a Lady with a Setter
Dog*, c. 1885. Oil on canvas, 30 × 23 in. The Metropolitan
Museum of Art, Fletcher Fund, 1933 (23.139).

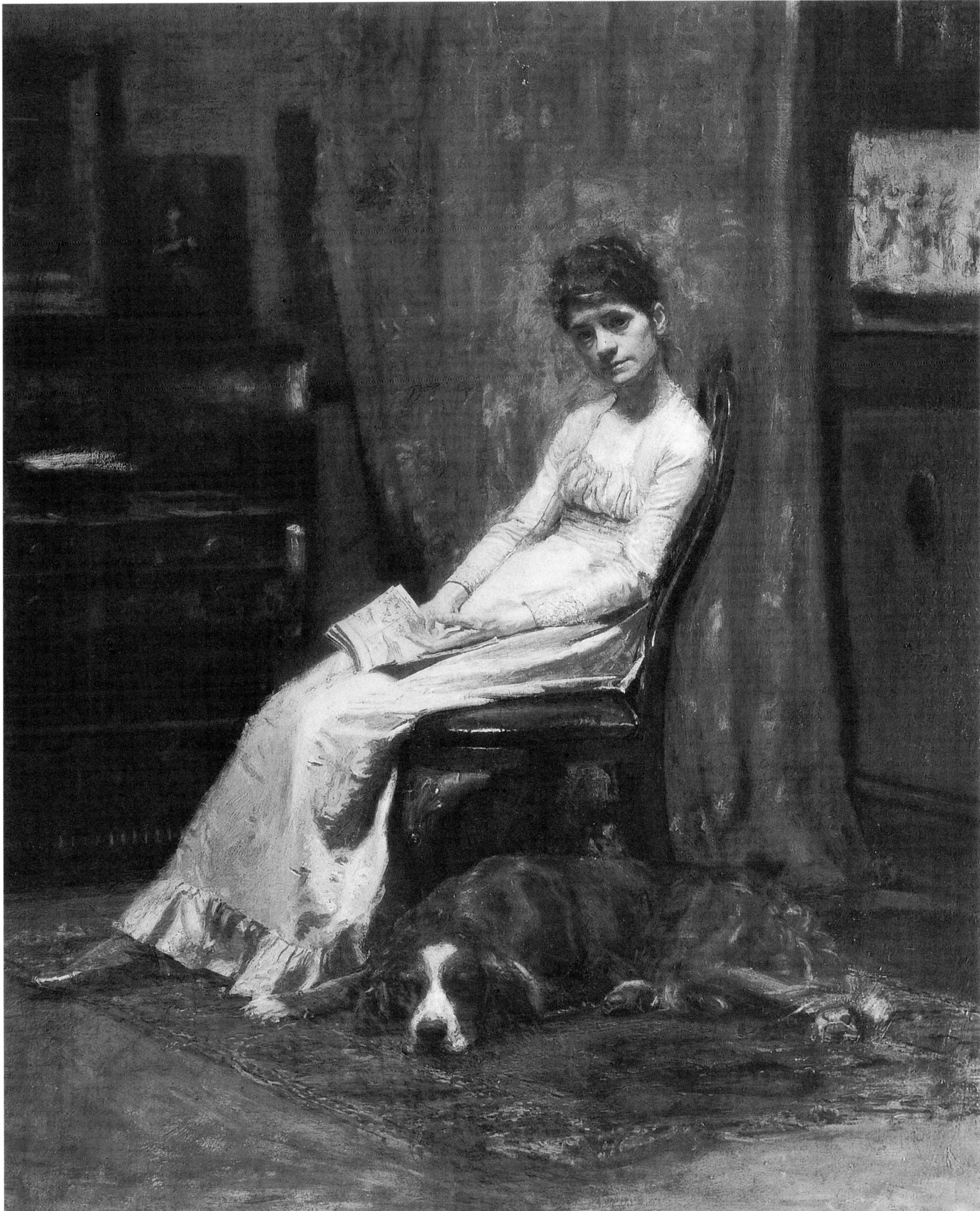

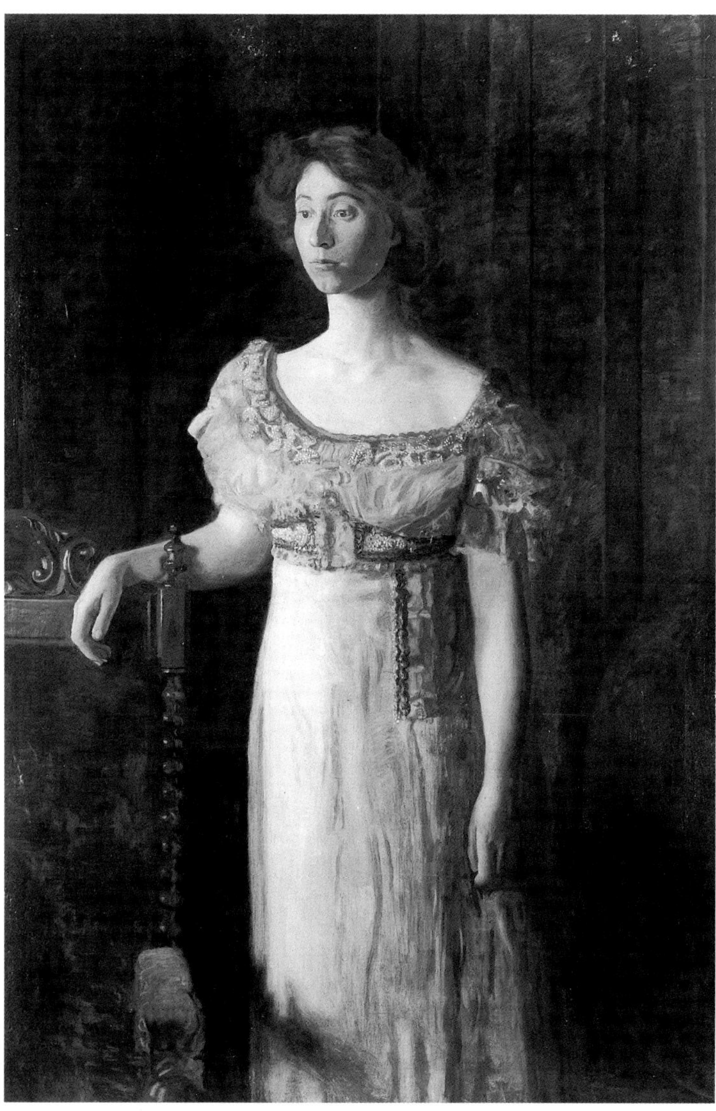

of Parker.[17] Though it is likely somewhat retouched, a publicity photo from around 1900, showing the smooth-complexioned actress Suzanne Santje in comparison with her wrinkled and heavy-featured appearance in Eakins's painting, is further evidence that the artist, far from being a simple recorder of facts, willingly transformed the realities in front of him.[18]

Eakins gained familiarity with the symptoms of female neurasthenia not only through his friendships with neurologists Horatio Wood and Mitchell, his interest in medicine, and the pervasiveness of neur-

asthenic representation in mass culture. Events in his personal life also contributed to his awareness of these signs of female nervousness and invalidism. First and foremost was the death of his mother. In June 1872, after two years of suffering and requiring constant care, Caroline Cowperthwait Eakins died from a recorded case of "exhaustion from mania."[19] Eakins had returned to Philadelphia in June 1870 to live with his parents after four years of study in Europe, and he would have been present to witness the entirety of his mother's decline. The premature deaths of three other loved ones likely added to his sense of women as unstable and unpredictable, prone to illness, and weak. In 1879, his fiancée, Kathrin Crowell, died of meningitis. Only three years later, his favorite sister, Margaret, who had the burden of managing the household after his mother's death, died from typhoid at age twenty-nine. Although she was shown in photographs as active and sporty and remembered by her nieces as a fun-loving aunt and a "grand person,"[20] the energetic aspects of Margaret's personality are not revealed in Eakins's portraits of his sister, *Margaret* and *Margaret in Skating Costume* (both c. 1871). Instead, the artist uses the formal elements found in his other portraits of women—bust format, tilted head, downcast gaze, harsh lighting—to portray his sister as brooding and wearied beyond her years. Six years after Margaret's death, Eakins's youngest sister, Caroline, died in 1889 at the age of twenty-four. She and her brother had not yet made amends over a feud that began three years earlier when Caroline heard about the indecent behavior of which Eakins was accused—sexual relations not only with his female students but also with their sister Margaret. From 1888 to 1892 a close friend and former student, Lilian Hammitt, sent Eakins a series of love letters discussing their upcoming marriage and his anticipated divorce from Susan; Eakins responded that she was "laboring under false notions," excusing her plans as a "mental disorder" and, later, as a "form of insanity."[21] Ultimately, Hammitt was put into a hospital. Though some claimed she was not insane, in Eakins's mind this was yet another encounter with an unstable, nervous female.[22] Finally, Ella Crowell, Eakins's seventeen-year-old niece who aspired to become an artist, came to live with Susan and him in

1890. She was committed to a hospital in 1896 and ended her life soon after. Ella's father had accused Eakins of corrupting, disturbing, and perhaps molesting his daughter. He banished the artist from the family farm at Avondale and forbade him contact with his nine other nephews and nieces—a result that would have confirmed for Eakins that the sick female was an especially troublesome figure.[23]

In light of such biographical issues, motivations for Eakins to paint the female neurasthenic become readily apparent. Around the time of his mother's death he began his excessively detailed perspective studies for his series of paintings showing rowers on the Schuylkill, perhaps expressing a sort of obsessive need to control the uncontrollable—nature, woman, illness, and death. The public's continual lack of acceptance of him and his art, the scandals in which he may have been unjustly accused, and his forced resignation from the Pennsylvania Academy would all have contributed to this need for regulation and mastery. As with the perspective studies, depictions of women with signs of neurasthenia functioned to fulfill this need: not only might they have quelled any guilt he may have felt for causing or not preventing their illnesses,[24] but they also would have lessened the women's threat to Eakins, whether this be the damaging of his reputation, the unjust blame and ostracism by living relatives, the pain caused by the women's introspection and death, or their potential challenge to male power and traditional gender roles.

The desire for self-control was also a likely impetus for producing these paintings. This applies both to the artist's alleged homosexual desires and to his status as a recovering neurasthenic—identities often conflated in the public mind. Physicians promoted self-restraint, control, and emotional detachment as a means of coping with the ever-present potential death of loved ones and decreasing the chance of nervousness.[25] As historian G. J. Barker-Benfield and others have noted, such demands for self-control were "often translated into a need to control women and resist their civilizing influences."[26] While the artist's manly "camp cure" out West allowed him an immediate escape from these feminine, "civilizing influences," Eakins's career-long representation of the female neurasthenic acted as

continued self-therapy through the transference of controlled object from the self to the nervous woman.[27] Further, this figure provided an "even less vigorous yardstick,"[28] one even more feminine and emotional, by which to judge himself.

In compliance with the troubling female presences in Eakins's own life, pervasive cultural concepts of the female invalid also influenced the artist's perceptions of the neurasthenic woman. In literature, popular magazines, and medical studies, female neurasthenics were represented as conniving, power-hungry, sympathy-craving, passive-aggressive creatures who endangered innocent lovers and husbands or impressionable younger women.[29] Although neurasthenia was commonly associated with the socially aberrant or intellectually ambitious woman, the neurasthenic as mother was considered particularly harmful. This may be another reason why Eakins did not depict woman as mother, though his sitters were certainly in the likely age group. While a healthy mother embodied self-sacrifice, the sick mother abandoned her duties and selfishly focused attention on her own ailments, jeopardizing the well-being of innocent family and friends who previously had depended on her. This configuration of the neurasthenic held particular significance for Eakins, considering that his invalid mother died early in his career, that his career was one of continual failure, and that the artist himself had a bout with neurasthenia.[30] The invalid mother was detrimental to the well-being of her whole family, but she held a special threat to the development of masculine traits in her son through her "demoralizing" and feminizing influences.[31]

In many cases—in Eakins's painting and in the wider culture—the danger posed by the neurasthenic woman commingled with her status as desired object, a combination derived from her association with "essential" womanhood and the dichotomies this concept incorporated throughout the nineteenth century. The state of illness not only exaggerated the contradictory roles of women as angelic martyr and evil temptress but also encompassed them both.[32] For the artist and his culture, emphasizing the female neurasthenic as sexual object expressed this simultaneous desire and threat; the fantasy of sexual possession served a metonymic function in which it stood as a substitute for a more general and complete control over and knowledge of the neurasthenic. The disheveled hair and clothes of many of Eakins's female sitters, while showing a distaste for the feminine and refined, also alluded to the sexual, as do these sitters' submissive, averted gazes. Medicine's treatment of the sick woman firmly established her erotic quality. Case descriptions of female patients often used sexual language, such as "an erotic tinge may be observable in her manner"[33] or Mitchell's suggestive "Too weak for wholesome restraint, she yields."[34] In his widely popular lecture demonstrations, Jean-Martin Charcot, as the master doctor, pushed buttonlike "hysterogenic," or ultra-sensitive, points on the patient's body to induce a convulsive, orgasmic hysteric fit. Whether viewed as a monster to be tamed, or as innocent, childlike, and vulnerable, the eroticized sick woman was customary in the arts as well. In Tony Robert-Fleury's 1878 painting, *Pinel Freeing the Madwomen*,[35] the patients rip open their blouses to expose their breasts, kneel, kiss men's hands, and willingly render themselves defenseless against the men's visual inspection of their bodies.[36]

Given the much more ambivalent feelings about male sickness and the biologically grounded association of women and illness, it is not surprising that indications of neurasthenia in Eakins's portraits of men are infrequent, ambiguous, and indirect. Whereas the female sitters are passive, emotional, and, in nearly all cases, confined to the interior, the artist depicts men as thinkers and doers, actively pursuing their specialty in the office or the outdoors; the teary eyes, vacant stares, and dimpled chins used to indicate neurasthenia in the portraits of women are nearly absent here. In this and in his reluctance to show men and women in the same painting, Eakins subscribed to the prevalent gender ideology of "separate spheres." In those few paintings that depict men and women together, such as *The Gross Clinic* (1875) and *The Agnew Clinic*, the contrast of the sexes is heightened through comparison: the women are passive and emotional, the men active and collected.[37]

Among the portraits of men alone, the most explicitly laudatory are the sporting scenes[38] and the *portraits d'apparat*, or those showing professionals in their work

environment. In the latter, for example, *Professor William D. Marks* (1886), the men are typically shown seated at their desks, at the site of their intellectual creativity and in the midst of work. They are surrounded by their inventions, tools of the trade, or masses of books—all material evidence and verification of their productivity (as opposed to Eakins's childless women) and intellectual capacity. In contrast to the paintings of seated women who slouch or lean back in their chairs, these men sit assured and confident and often lean forward with their forearms on the desk, their hands holding a pencil or keeping a place in a book. Intersecting diagonals and straight lines give action and vibrancy to the canvases, in striking contrast to the drooping lines of *The Actress* or *Lady with a Setter Dog*. In others, masculine signs of activity, intelligence, and professional standing are more subtle, whether simply the held piece of paper in *Professor Leslie Miller* (1901) or the robed attire of the figure in *The Dean's Roll Call* (1899) or, in both cases, the title. Even in the bust portraits, the men are usually shown with brows crinkled in thought, gazes confronting the viewer, heads held upright, and direct frontal or impersonal profile poses. Unlike the blank stares, averted gazes, tilted heads, and three-quarter turn commonly found in the portraits of women, these iconographic elements deemphasize any emotional content.[39]

Nonetheless, neurasthenia is occasionally indicated in Eakins's portraits of men. While these signs at first appear to be entirely absent from the *portraits d'apparat*, the sloped shoulders and downcast gaze in *Frank Hamilton Cushing*,[40] for example, or the red-rimmed eyes of *Professor Henry Rowland* (1897) suggest otherwise. Such elements seem incongruous with the portraits' overall emotional reticence and the abundant signs of the sitters' professional successes (such as the Zuni artifacts surrounding the anthropologist Cushing, or Rowland's invention and claim to fame, the spectroscope, prominently displayed in the scientist's hand). However, the subtle suggestions of weariness gain meaning and clarity when read in the context of period discussions of male nervousness. Physicians specializing in this area often downplayed the emotional excess so crucial to the diagnosis of female neurasthenia. Beard, for example, made it

clear that "nervousness does not mean . . . a predomi-
nance of the emotional, with a relative inferiority of
intellectual nature." He even invented a term to distin-
guish nervousness in professionals from that found in
bored housewives: "cerebrasthenia," or brain neurasthenia. Further, unlike the biological cause of neurasthenia
in women, overwork was cited as the main cause of nervousness in men, thus emphasizing this state as exceptional rather than as natural and normal. Through
showing mental and physical exhaustion, rather than
emotional strain, Eakins best communicated the "distin-
guished malady" that afflicted these male professionals.[41]

For nineteenth-century viewers of these portraits,
neurasthenic traits would add to, rather than subtract
from, the overall heroic tone, particularly in the context
of other valorizing iconography. In men, the illness
could signal intelligence and fulfillment of duty, determination, and success in their careers—all evidence of
virile manhood—while also serving as a badge of their
martyrdom and dedication to the progress of the race
and nation. Some believed that male neurasthenics
were the "superior individuals, the scholars, poets
and statesmen" who, physician Mary Putnam Jacobi
claimed, "were ready to sacrifice their health for higher
goals."[42] Thus, the artist's insistence that Professor
Miller wear an old jacket and Dean Holland old shoes
(which still identify them as professionals)[43] could have
been an effort to symbolize, in Mitchell's terms, this
"wear and tear"[44] due to overwork as well as a disregard
for material appearance in a whirlwind of intellectual
creativity. However, while celebrating "higher goals" and
social progress, these portraits also seem to share with
Eakins's Arcadian paintings and nostalgic historical
works[45] reservations about the advent of modernity,
believed by some physicians to be the cause of nervousness.[46] By showing that the illness could afflict the leading American thinkers and producers, Eakins may have
been revealing what he felt was a crisis in the nation:
the approaching downfall of the caretakers of society,
and thus of advanced society itself.[47]

Although the advent of cerebrasthenia allowed men
to be ill and retain a sense of masculinity, this state of
illness had a long history as one of weakness and thus,
as mentioned, as one closely associated with women.[48]

While the woman became like the "unschooled child"
when afflicted with neurasthenia, Mitchell believed that
when nervous "the strong man becomes like the average
woman."[49] In this sense, then, even as neurasthenia was
seen as a sign of manly success and intellect and its cure
an indication of strong will, it continued to carry the
stigma of failure and weakness for succumbing to emotions and malady in the first place.[50] If neither overwork
nor an unusual, traumatic occurrence could be cited as
the cause, doctors were quick to note their male patient
was "a delicate looking man" with a "peculiar constitution."[51] Perhaps it was this ambiguous relation between
neurasthenia and men—on the one hand a sign of
heroism, on the other a sign of effeminacy—that kept
Eakins from more frequently showing signs of nervousness in his *portraits d'apparat*.

A handful of emotionally charged anomalies among
Eakins's portraits of men include more explicit and
more feminine signs of neurasthenia. Hardly heroiciz-
ing, these paintings bear striking similarities to the formal, iconographic, and emotional content of Eakins's
portraits of women; the artist presents the teary-eyed
sitters in sharply dramatic lighting, at a three-quarter
angle, and with tilted heads and downcast or vacant
gazes. With the exception of the self-portraits, these
works portray youths: three of Eakins's own students
(*Samuel Murray* from 1889, *Francis Ziegler* from 1890, and
Portrait of Douglass M. Hall [fig. 26]) and one of a musi-
cian, *The Pianist* (1896). With their clear, neurasthenic
signs of emotional instability and their effeminizing
iconography, the portraits of the young men could indicate the artist's wish to show the inner conflict and
trauma of youth, of passing into an unsure, demanding
world of adulthood, of coping with a burgeoning sexuality. Representing these young men with signs of
neurasthenia only further communicated their liminal
status of passage. Contemporary thought on nervous
illness held that young men, like all women, were especially susceptible to neurasthenia and emotional breakdowns caused by the stress and strains of the demands
of adulthood. Significantly, all four young men were
artists (like Eakins), and the general pressure to gain
manly success in their careers was magnified by that
potentially feminine profession, adding to the already

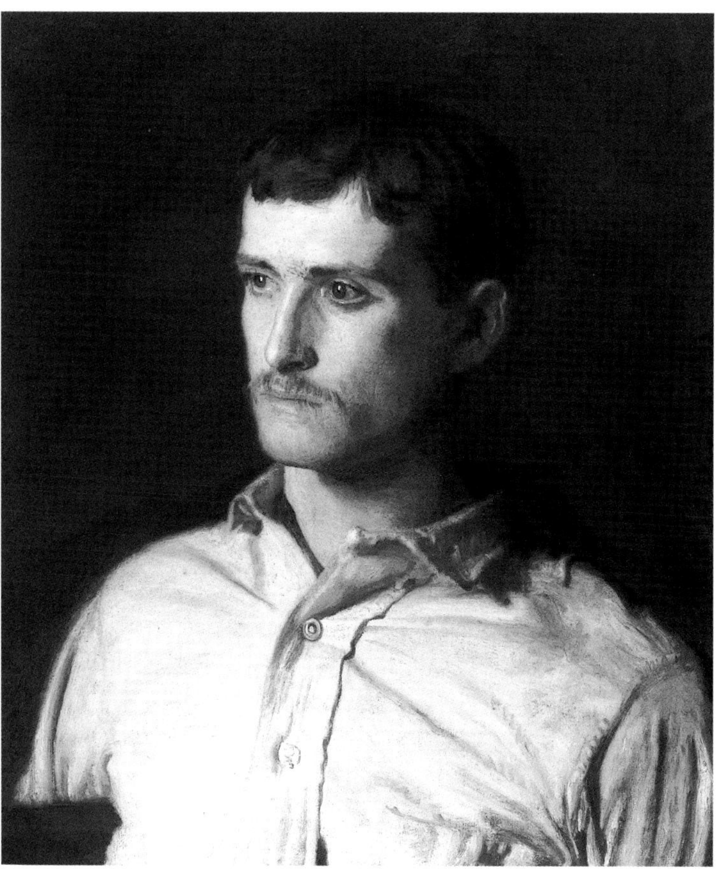

FIG. 26 Thomas Eakins, *Portrait of Douglass M. Hall*, c. 1888. Oil on canvas, 24½ × 20½ in. Philadelphia Museum of Art. Given by Mrs. William E. Studdiford.

high gender conflict of youth.[52] In *Portrait of Douglass M. Hall*, especially, a melancholy tone accompanies signs of developing sexuality—the visible though somewhat sparse mustache, the strong jawline, and the breadth of shoulders and muscularity, which, judging by the taut lines of the sitter's shirt, were only recently acquired.

Eakins's own experience of young manhood supports this interpretation. Victorian America experienced a widespread gender crisis and questioning of sexual identity, and the artist had a number of personal "failings" in the early 1870s. As Martin Berger notes, Eakins "bought his way out of Civil War service, was unmarried, lived and worked in his parents' home, was engaged in a profession that had long held effeminate associations, and was unable to earn his own living." He had, "in other words, failed to achieve a number of important 'milestones' of manhood."[53] Berger looks to the rowing pictures—with their explicit display of

unquestionable masculinity not only in their emphasis on physical musculature and prowess, but also in the attention paid to the outdoors and wide open spaces and to such themes as determination and hard work—as evidence of, and an attempt to compensate for, the artist's gender insecurities. Though not as obviously masculine as the rowing pictures, the portraits of the four young men would have served as compensation as well. Portraying these sitters as emotionally distressed and vulnerable allowed Eakins to normalize his own experience; the insecurities he had as a young man are divorced from his personal failings and become, rather, an intrinsic part of the initiation into manhood.

Secondly, these portraits present homoerotic images, functioning for Eakins as a sort of fantasy, a means to sexual domination through images of young men's emotional and sexual vulnerability. The portraits have been described by one scholar as "romantic" and "sensual"—hardly the adjectives one would use in conjunction with the paintings of middle-aged intellectuals.[54] Indeed, in comparison with the bulk of depictions of men, these youths are quite feminized and sexualized.[55] While this reading may partially be inspired by the sitters' rather boyish faces and curly hair, the artist obviously emphasized certain elements. Through lighting, pose, and the close-up, bust format, Eakins accentuated lush lashes and full, curving lips, or fluffy, bright-pink bow ties, contributing to the overall designation of these sitters as effeminate sex objects.

Homosexuality itself was commonly considered a form of illness. Contemporary articles on homosexuality, labeled "perverted sexuality" and "sodomy," were published in medical journals on both nervous and physical disease, thus identifying homosexuality as an unhealthy state that needed to be cured.[56] The converse was also true—neurasthenia could be a sign of homosexuality or effeminacy. Medical studies often noted the male neurasthenic's thin, anemic appearance and lack of manly musculature.[57] French physician Jean Martin Charcot explained male hysterics by claiming that they were unusually "effeminate,"[58] and, more scornfully, Emile Batault in 1885 wrote that hysterical men were "timid and fearful men. . . . Coquettish and eccentric, they prefer ribbons and scarves to hard manual labor."

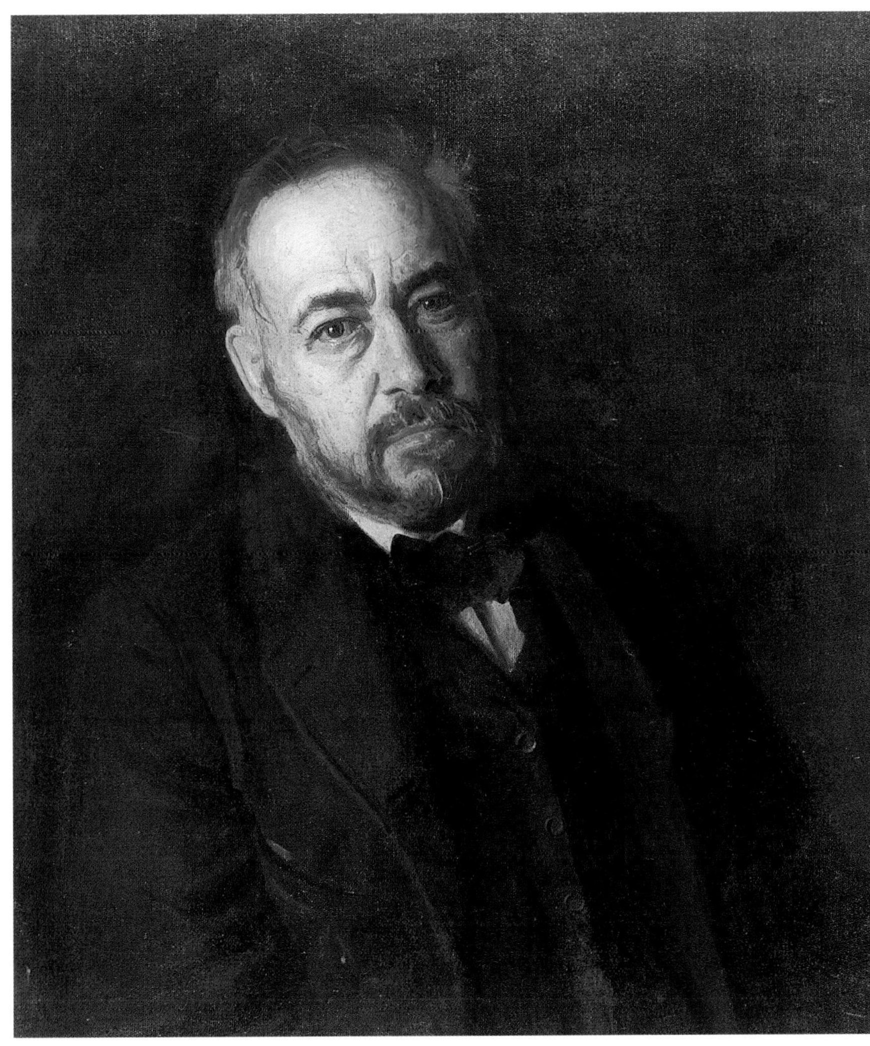

Other physicians actually noted that these men were homosexual.[59] With his four portraits, as with the Arcadia scenes and *Swimming Hole* (c. 1883–85), Eakins may have been taking a nostalgic look back to youth[60] when homosocial and even homoerotic desire was considered normal. In tracing a number of intimate letters between young male friends who addressed each other more like lovers, Anthony Rotondo finds that "in young manhood, romantic—even passionate—friendships between males were socially accepted."[61] However, for a married, working man, the romance and carefree play of youth were set aside: "Friendship did not disappear from the lives of mature men, but it never regained the passionate intensity of youth."[62] While the artist's relationships with his students have long been a point of speculation,[63] the point is not to claim that the artist was homosexual, though this may well have been the case, but to suggest that he indeed felt some sort of tension between homosexual desire and anxiety, and he may have used his canvases as a site to work out, consciously or not, this fantasy and tension.[64]

The only other works that show such conspicuous signs of emotional trauma are the pair of self-portraits completed in 1902. In the first, an unfinished, closely cropped image, the artist peers out at the viewer with a cocked eyebrow. Combined with the dark colors, dramatic lighting, and violent brush strokes, these elements give the work a sinister tone; the artist appears vengeful and angry, even mentally unsound. In the other (fig. 27), a completed work, Eakins posed himself in a role that is not as directly threatening. Using a less imposing, slightly larger format, he shows himself with a tilted head, mussed hair, teary eyes, and a frowning mouth, accentuated by the sloping line of his mustache.

Such iconographic elements clearly affiliate this work with his portraits of women and the several young men. Unlike these prototypes, however, his emotional, "troubled" look is combined with a confrontational, questioning gaze. The result is a painting that readily evokes sympathy from the viewer yet also maintains the accusatory tone of the first self-portrait.

Eakins chose to depict himself with the more explicitly neurasthenic iconography of his portraits of emotional women rather than in the usual format he used to show men as intellectual heroes. Both self-portraits were in response to the requirement for associate membership into the National Academy. After roughly thirty years of neglect and lack of appreciation from the academy, the membership must have seemed a mere token offering, and the artist may have used these self-portraits to communicate his bitterness and scorn.[65] In the evolution of the self-portraits, he progressed from the overtly hostile and aggressive tone in the sketch (perhaps a way to vent some preliminary anger) to the more clever, passive-aggressive device in the finished painting. Rather than turning members of the academy away through threat, the latter painting may have been intended to evoke guilt for not recognizing the artist earlier and thus preventing his emotional weariness.

Eakins indeed promoted himself as the isolated, underappreciated genius, the overworked intellectual; his use of distinct neurasthenic signs in his finished self-portrait only aided in communicating this status. His 1894 statement stands as just one of many pieces of evidence: "My honors are misunderstanding, persecution, and neglect, enhanced because unsought."[66] Contrasting the cosmopolitanism suggested by William Merritt Chase's atelier, Eakins left his studio undecorated and messy, with signs of activity everywhere—casts, photographs, works in progress, notes to himself simply written on the wall—giving the message to all who entered that he was constantly in a whirlwind of creative mental activity, similar to the intellectual heroes whom he portrayed with open books scattered across their desks. Analogous to the studio was his unkempt appearance—yet another indication of neurasthenic status—represented in the final self-portrait by his

mussed hair and unevenly trimmed mustache. Combined with his reputation as extra-sensitive and emotional (he was known to have cried at musical performances),[67] such physical disarray draws upon mythical notions of the artist as gifted seer, as underappreciated because he is ahead of his time, as a mad genius obsessive about his creations and constantly at work. It also works on the notion of the godlike androgyny of genius, in which emotional tendencies translate into enhanced perception. Not surprisingly, the concept of the artist as mad genius entered into nineteenth-century theories of neurosis. One vivid example is Dr. Jacques-Joseph Moreau's (1804–1884) "tree of nervosity," in which each branch divides nervous illnesses into types, one branch reserved specifically for "exceptional intelligence" and with a special sub-branch labeled "Arts."[68] In addition, neurasthenia was epidemic among cultural producers and leaders of the time. Those afflicted include both Beard and Mitchell, Theodore Roosevelt, Thorstein Veblen, Jane Addams, Edith Wharton, Jack London, Theodore Dreiser, and William and Henry James, among a long list of others.[69] By depicting himself as explicitly neurasthenic and as possessing an otherwise "feminine" sensitivity, Eakins claimed his status among this prestigious group and, undeniably, marked himself as the overworked, misunderstood genius, fully deserving the honors that came all too late.[70]

In all its forms—the sexualized, deceptive temptress, the selfish mother, or the rebellious feminist; the heroic intellectual, the troubled effeminate youth, or the mad genius—neurasthenia provided for Eakins what it did for much of late nineteenth-century America: a magnifier of already present realities and myths, an answer to questions, a definition that embraced contradictions intact that were otherwise incoherent and impossible to unify. On a personal, psychological level, figuring the neurasthenic functioned for Eakins as a means of expressing and controlling the anxiety and tension within himself and his sexuality, his identity as a neurasthenic, and his problematic relationships with nervous women. For us, reinscribing the neurasthenic onto his portraits both clarifies their ambiguity and, at the same time, retains it. The reinscription explains the worn appearance of many sitters and the divergent messages and interpretations of their weariness, but this explanation is nuanced and multifaceted, acknowledging the very real complexities and contradictions of the paintings, of their surrounding culture, and of the artist that produced them.

Notes

This essay is reprinted with permission and slight revisions from *Nineteenth-Century Studies* 12 (1998): 84–109.

1. Sylvan Schendler, *Eakins* (Boston: Little, Brown & Co., 1967), 145.

2. William J. Clark, "The Iconography of Gender in Thomas Eakins Portraiture," *American Studies* 32, no. 2 (Fall 1991): 17, 21.

3. Schendler, 138.

4. Other researchers who have mentioned a possible connection between Eakins's portraits and neurasthenia are Lifton, Johns, Clark, and Lutz. Lifton makes considerable contributions to discussions of the similarities of the careers of and the personal relationship between the neurologist Mitchell and Eakins. The latter three explorations are more brief. See Norma Lifton, "Thomas Eakins and S. Weir Mitchell: Images in Cures in the Late Nineteenth Century," *Psychoanalytic Perspectives on Art* 2 (1987); Elizabeth Johns, *Thomas Eakins: The Heroism of Modern Life* (Princeton, NJ: Princeton University Press, 1983); and Tom Lutz, *American Nervousness, 1903: An Anecdotal History* (Ithaca, NY: Cornell University Press, 1991).

5. Francis G. Gosling, *Before Freud: Neurasthenia and the American Medical Community, 1870–1910* (Urbana: University of Illinois Press, 1987), 50, 78–79.

6. Lutz, 2, 217.

7. For more background on neurasthenia, see Gosling, and George Frederick Drinka, *The Birth of Neurosis: Myth, Malady and the Victorians* (New York: Simon and Schuster, 1984); in relation to gender, see Diane Price Herndl, *Invalid Women: Figuring Feminine Illness in American Fiction and Culture, 1840–1940* (Chapel Hill: University of North Carolina Press, 1993), and Anthony E. Rotondo, *American Manhood: Transformations in Masculinity from the Revolution to the Modern Era* (New York: Basic Books, 1993). For contemporary sources, see George M. Beard, *American Nervousness: Its Causes and Consequences* (New York: G. P. Putnam's Sons, 1881); S. Weir Mitchell, "Clinical Lecture on Nervousness in the Male," *The Medical News and Library* 35 (December 1877): 177–84; Mitchell, *Doctor and Patient* (Philadelphia: J. B. Lippincott & Co., 1888); and Mitchell, *Fat and Blood: An Essay on the Treatment of Certain Forms of Neurasthenia and Hysteria* (London: J. B. Lippincott & Co., 1891).

8. Mitchell, *Doctor and Patient*, 10.

9. Ellwood C. Parry, "The Thomas Eakins Portrait of Sue and Harry: Or, When Did the Artist Change His Mind?" *Arts Magazine* 53, no. 9 (May 1979): 146–53.

10. Mitchell, *Fat and Blood*, 30.

11. Carroll Smith-Rosenberg, *Disorderly Conduct: Visions of Gender in Victorian America* (New York: Alfred A. Knopf, 1985), 190–91.

12. Bram Dijkstra, *Idols of Perversity: Fantasies of Feminine Evil in Fin-de-Siècle Culture* (New York: Oxford University Press, 1986), 43.

13. Generally, the awkwardness of this and other portraits has been attributed to the fact that the artist did not know the sitter. However, Eakins and Greenewalt were, in fact, friends. See Lloyd Goodrich, "About a Man Who Did Not Care to Be Written About: Portraits in Friendship of Thomas Eakins," *Arts Magazine* 53, 9 (May 1979): 96–100.

14. Gosling, 48; Mitchell, *Doctor and Patient*, 120.

15. Smith-Rosenberg, 206.

16. Another photo of the sitter, also dated c. 1891 (Olympia Galleries, Philadelphia), gives Van Buren a more hollowed face, thus indeed looking more like her aged appearance in the portrait. Van Buren is one of the few female sitters who we know suffered from a chronic illness, periodically having to leave Philadelphia for treatment in Detroit. The nature of this illness, its treatment, and its time span are all unknown. If Van Buren did show signs of aging, depression, and illness at the time of Eakins's portrait, the artist only exaggerated these features through methods of lighting, pose, and diminution of the figure by placing her in a large, bulky chair.

17. Gordon Hendricks, *The Photographs of Thomas Eakins* (New York: Grossman, 1972).

18. In addition to such alterations, Eakins was also disinclined to represent certain figures altogether. Although the opportunity to show women as active, outdoors, or heroic in duty was not as prevalent then as now, it is incorrect to think that Eakins had no other option than to depict women as passive, emotional, and confined to the interior. Hendricks points out that photographs by the artist of women horseback riding or swimming show precisely how disinclined he was to incorporate these images of activity into his paintings of women. Considering that Eakins preferred to adhere to roles that better complied with the prevailing traditional thoughts on gender, it seems striking that he did not once depict woman as mother. The absence appears particularly odd since he took so many photographs of Frances, Margaret, and Susan with children; see Gordon Hendricks, *The Life and Work of Thomas Eakins* (New York: Grossman Publishers, 1974). The subject was one that could easily have been heroicized, comparable to the images of male leaders he chose to depict. As motherhood represented healthy, functioning womanhood and, further, was sometimes seen as a cure for sickness, the lack of the mother figure in his

paintings may have been an additional way for Eakins to indicate woman's illness.

19. Lloyd Goodrich, *Thomas Eakins*, 2 vols. (Cambridge, MA:
Harvard University Press, 1982).

20. Margaret McHenry, *Thomas Eakins, Who Painted*
(Oreland, PA: M. McHenry, 1946), 95.

21. Kathleen Foster and Cheryl Liebold, *Writing About
Eakins* (Philadelphia: University of Pennsylvania Press, 1989),
98, 99n. 9.

22. Given their friendship and Eakins's paternalistic mone-
tary and emotional support of Hammitt, he may have felt that
he could have done more to help Hammitt, or that he had
somehow been the cause of her illness by misleading her about
his intentions and feelings.

23. The troublesome nature of Eakins's personal relations
with females often manifested itself in his seemingly hostile and
condescending treatment of the opposite sex. Such behavior
included the artist's touching and poking of his sitters' breasts,
persistently urging them to pose nude (Hendricks, *The Photographs of Thomas Eakins*), exposing his naked body to a young
model, using "feminine" as a derogatory adjective, and making
such comments as "I do not believe that the great painting or
sculpture or surgery will ever be done by women" (Foster and
Liebold, 139n. 9, 236). For more on Eakins's relationships with
women, see also Goodrich, and William Innes Homer, *Thomas
Eakins: His Life and Art* (New York: Abbeville Press, 1992), 179.

24. Whether he felt this guilt or not, he was still accused of
fault in the case of Ella Crowell and Lilian Hammitt, and it is
likely that these accusations may have had some effect on him.

25. Barbara Sicherman, "The Paradox of Prudence: Mental
Health in the Gilded Age," *The Journal of American History* 62,
4 (March 1976): 890–912.

26. Herndl, 80.

27. Whereas inactivity, dependence, and domesticity defined
the rest cure for women, the men often underwent the camp or
exercise cure, which prescribed large amounts of activity and
outdoor excursions. See Roy Porter, "The Body and the Mind,
the Doctor and the Patient," in *Hysteria Beyond Freud*, ed. Sander
L. Gilman et al. (Berkeley: University of California Press, 1993),
225–85, and Lutz, 32. On the male desire to control and resist
the female civilizing influence, see G. J. Barker-Benfield, *The
Horrors of the Half-Known Life: Male Attitudes Toward Women and
Sexuality in Nineteenth-Century America* (New York: Harper &
Row, 1976), 3–61, and Rotondo, 232–46.

28. Barker-Benfield, 258.

29. See David Rein, *S. Weir Mitchell as a Psychiatric Novelist*
(New York: International Universities Press, 1952).

30. With the theory that nervous strength could be inher-
ited, "parents were held accountable for 'husbanding' their own
nervous energy so that their children would not be handicapped
in the race of life" (Gosling, 88).

31. In the very act of painting, Eakins was able to limit the
actions and emotions of his subjects and avoid the extremities
of neurosis (the torrents of tears, the uncontrollable, seizure-like
"fits"). By eternally preserving the ill woman on canvas and turning her image literally into an aesthetic object, Eakins could gain
the detachment suggested by physicians and stave off the emotional pain of her death. Repeatedly painting his female sitters'
gaze as indirect and away from himself, as seen in *Alice Kurtz*
and *Addie*, among others, was yet another means of solidifying
his control and averting the neurasthenic's potential harm.

32. Also see Oliver Wendell Holmes, quoted in Smith-
Rosenberg, 207; and also Drinka, 202, and Rein, 103–4.

33. Porter, in Gilman, *Hysteria Beyond Freud*, 254.

34. Mitchell, *Doctor and Patient*, 119.

35. An 1887 painting by André Brouillet (like Eakins, a student of Gérôme's) of Charcot's lecture hall shows the neurotic
female, vulnerable and acquiescent in her fainting, further sexualized by her loose, fallen blouse.

36. Some scholars have suggested that Eakins was expressing
a form of sympathy for, or even empathy with, women through
the production of these works, providing a sort of feminist cri-
tique of patriarchy (Clark, "Iconography of Gender," 6, 26). However, given the prevailing gender ideology as well as the difference
in cures and connotations of his illness as a man, this sympathy
could only have been a patronizing one, much like the "pitying
patronage" and "condescending tenderness" that male physicians
felt toward their female patients (Golden et al., 111, 116; Mitchell,
Doctor and Patient, 11). Though Eakins certainly had the ability to
criticize his surrounding culture, to endow him with such great
powers of sympathy is to see him as transcending his own time
and gender role to achieve the mythical identity of the artist as a
gifted seer, a neutral and omniscient genius.

37. For more in-depth treatment of gender in the *Clinic* paintings, see, for example, Diana E. Long, "The Medical World of *The
Agnew Clinic*: A World We Have Lost," *Prospects* 11 (1987): 185–98;
or Judith Fryer, "The Body in Pain in Thomas Eakins' *Agnew
Clinic*," *Michigan Quarterly Review* 30 (Winter 1991): 191–209.

38. For a thorough discussion of the rowing paintings and
their heroic element, see Elizabeth Johns, "*Max Schmitt in a Single
Scull* or *The Champion Single Sculls*," in Schendler, *Eakins*.

39. For examples of such iconography in Eakins's portraits of
men, see *Frank Linton* (1904), *William Merritt Chase* (1899), and
Henry O. Tanner (1902).

40. According to William Truettner ("Dressing the Part:
Thomas Eakins' *Portrait of Frank Hamilton Cushing*," *American Art
Journal* 17 [Spring 1985]: 48–72), Cushing's four-and-a-half-year
stay (a few years prior to this portrait) in the Southwest to
study the Zuni culture ruined his health and resulted in his suffering bouts of anxiety regarding his cultural identity (50–52).
Perhaps these individual stories account for the appearance of
neurasthenia in the portraits of men.

41. George M. Beard, quoted in Lutz, 6.

42. Sicherman, 911.

43. Hendricks, *The Photographs of Thomas Eakins*, 250.

44. Mitchell, *Wear and Tear; or, Hints for the Overworked* (London: J. B. Lippincott & Co., 1871).

45. See, for example, Eakins's painting *In Grandmother's Time* (1876).

46. Gosling, 90.

47. For more on the work ethic of Victorian manhood, see Rotondo. Others, such as George M. Beard, also expressed "fear of the possible degeneration of the handful of people who are the caretakers of a fragile civilization," cited in Lutz, 7.

48. Even the mad genius myth, while almost exclusively associated with illness in men, was designated for the unusual, those extra-sensitive gifted artists and thinkers who were so above others as to, like God, combine traits of both sexes.

49. Mitchell, "Clinical Lecture on Nervousness in the Male," 179.

50. See Lutz, and Rotondo, 222–46, for discussions of these differing attitudes toward male illness.

51. Mitchell, "Clinical Lecture on Nervousness in the Male," 182.

52. See Rotondo, 56–91, for more on young manhood, gender insecurities, and male compensation in the Victorian era.

53. Martin Berger, "Painting Victorian Manhood," in *Thomas Eakins: The Rowing Pictures*, exh. cat., Yale University Art Gallery, ed. Helen A. Cooper (New Haven: Yale University Press, 1996), 102–4.

54. Schendler, 111.

55. During this time, homosexuality was defined as specifically feminine; Beard said homosexuals were "men become women" (Rotondo, 276–77).

56. Whitney Davis, "Erotic Revision in Thomas Eakins's Narratives of Male Nudity," *Art History* 17, no. 3 (September 1994): 301–41. Davis cites the following examples: William Dickinson, "A Case of Sodomy," *St. Louis Medical and Surgical Journal* 40 (1881): 196–97 (which notes that anal intercourse is "frequently committed" among boys); G. Alder Blumer, "A Case of Perverted Sexual Instinct," *American Journal of Insanity* 39 (1882): 22–25; and J. C. Shaw and G. N. Ferris, "Perverted Sexual Instinct," *Journal of Nervous and Mental Disease* 10 (1883): 184–204. Davis is one of several scholars who have recently explored Eakins's relation to homosexuality.

57. Gosling, 39.

58. Drinka, 101.

59. Porter, in Gilman et. al., *Hysteria Beyond Freud*, 289.

60. That Whitney Davis, 330, has pointed out that some of the figures in the *Swimming Hole*, including Eakins himself, are far past their youth even further supports this scene as a sign of "escape," though temporary, from the adult world of responsibility and strict heterosexuality.

61. For a discussion of these letters, see Rotondo, 75–91.

62. Ibid., 7, 90–91.

63. It is well known that he formed close friendships with many of them, particularly with Samuel Murray. The two were said to have spent much time with one another and to have taken long trips together, and Murray did not get married until after Eakins's death. In addition, Eakins let only Murray feed him on his deathbed, refusing the offers of women, such as Addie and his wife, to do so (Hendricks, *Life and Work of Thomas Eakins*, 221–22, 276). The artist and his students often posed nude for each other, and though at first this may simply seem a typical act of economy and practicality, it gains additional meaning in this context.

64. A similar dynamic of conflict appears in other paintings by Eakins as well, namely *Salutat* and *The Swimming Hole*, in which the artist places homoerotic elements in the context of a safely masculine sporting atmosphere or the innocent boyhood world of play. See Davis, 315–18, 328, for more on the homoerotic elements of *The Swimming Hole*.

65. For other indications of the artist's bitterness, see Goodrich, 201. Darell Sewell also made this connection, though in a somewhat different context. See his entry on the portraits in *Thomas Eakins*, ed. John Wilmerding (Washington, D.C.: Smithsonian Institution Press, 1993). Although Eakins himself underwent a period of nervous exhaustion in 1886, these portraits were painted a full sixteen years later, and thus the experience seems an unlikely reason for the portraits' outcome. Lutz notes that neurasthenia was described by many period authors as "caused by a society with too strenuous a reaction to scandal and too disciplinary a reaction to scandalous desires" (52–55). It may have been such a critical statement on society's overreaction to scandal that Eakins was trying to communicate with the representation of himself as neurasthenic.

66. Goodrich, 160.

67. Elizabeth Johns, *American Genre Paintings: The Politics of Everyday Life* (New Haven: Yale University Press, 1991), 115.

68. Moreau, known as the creator of the "genius myth" as an explanation of neurosis, worked most of his life at the Bicetre, the counterpart for men of the Salpetrière, the famed Parisian hospital for female neurotics.

69. Lutz, 19.

70. These self-portraits, in their depiction of an overtly emotional artist suffering from inner turmoil, stand in a long tradition of artists' self-portraits—for example, some of those by Rembrandt and Courbet. This would further solidify the view that Eakins was trying to place himself within a tradition of "genius" artists.

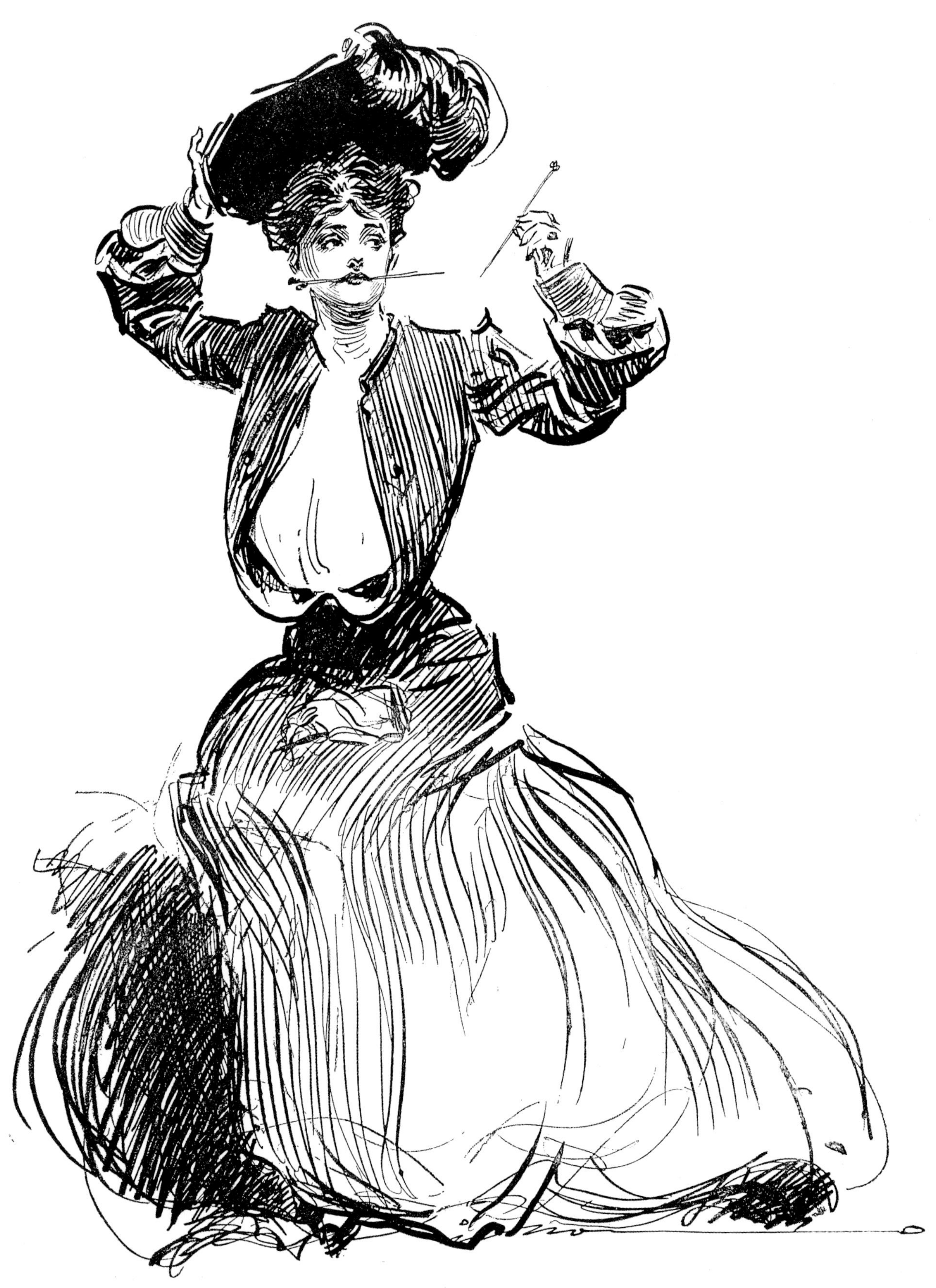

AMANDA GLESMANN

REFORMING THE LADY

CHARLES DANA GIBSON AND THE "NEW GIRL"

In 1901 two contemporary women encountered each other face-to-face in the pages of *The Atlantic Monthly*.[1] A four-page short story by Caroline Ticknor—published that July—imagined a passive, genteel, late-Victorian lady meeting the more youthful, spirited figure known as the Gibson Girl. Ticknor's "steel-engraving lady" was a familiar figure from steel-plate engravings like those used to illustrate fashion magazines such as *Godey's Lady's Book*. Like the passive, introspective Women at Home painted by Thomas Wilmer Dewing, she was a delicate creature who was usually posed indoors and often seemed on the verge of nervous exhaustion and collapse—a perfect candidate for neurasthenia.[2] The other type, the Gibson Girl, had circulated widely in drawings and illustrations since 1890, when she first appeared in *Life*, a popular humor magazine. She was a new, more modern and independent woman. She was strong and spirited, usually seen taking part in activities outside the home. Turn-of-the-century readers recognized the steel-engraving lady and the Gibson Girl as contrasting models of womanhood. Ticknor exaggerates their differences to the point of caricature, and the clash between them is hilarious. It is as difficult for the two to coexist in print as it was for actual women to

reconcile traditional female roles with the opportunities available to them in the late nineteenth century.

When Ticknor's story begins, we find the steel-engraving lady alone, dreamily awaiting her lover, Reginald. Her apartment is pervaded by "an air of quiet repose" and ornamented with the elaborate fancywork and embroidered mottoes a proper lady might be expected to produce. Suddenly, a heavy step is heard on the stairs. The steel-engraving lady expects Reginald, but when the door flies open it is the Gibson Girl who stands on the threshold facing her. The Gibson Girl is on her way to meet a friend at the golf course, but she explains that she has stopped by in order to research the steel-engraving lady for a paper she is writing on "extinct types." The lady remains unfailingly—and excessively—courteous to her guest but clearly disapproves of and is shocked by the Gibson Girl's strong, casual manner, sunburned skin, and practical clothing. When the irrepressible Gibson Girl announces that she

FIG. 28 [*facing*] Charles Dana Gibson, *Untitled (Gibson Girl Pinning Her Hat)*, 1904. This and the following images in this article were reproduced from *The Gibson Book: A Collection of the Published Works of Charles Dana Gibson* (New York: C. Scribner's Sons, 1906).

plans to pursue a professional life outside the home, it is clear that the divergence between the two figures is insurmountable.

Ticknor presents the Gibson Girl as a modern woman and the equal of men. She has a college education and, as she proudly asserts, she is not part of the "shy, retiring, uncomplaining generation" that came before her. She and her peers are "up to date and up to snuff, and every one of us is self-supporting." The steel-engraving lady, bewildered by such behavior, protests, "Your public aspirations, your independent views, your discontent, are something I cannot understand." As the story ends, the steel-engraving lady remains ensconced in her parlor, singing a "quaint old ballad" to Reginald, while the Gibson Girl moves out-of-doors and joins a young man for golf.

The steel-engraving lady, like the Woman at Home depicted by artists such as Dewing, John White Alexander, and Edmund Tarbell, was the quintessential genteel type idealized in the late Victorian period as a model wife and mother. The Gibson Girl was an entirely new figure. She was beautiful and flirtatious, spirited, confident, and yet unmistakably feminine. She was also active and healthy—notable characteristics at a time when neurasthenia had become an all too common affliction. When she threw open the door to the steel-engraving lady's apartment she directly challenged the limits of the genteel woman's confining domestic world.

From the moment the Gibson Girl arrived on the pages of weekly journals in 1890 she became a popular fixture in the American imagination.[3] By the time Ticknor's story was published she could be found in *Life*, *The Century*, *Collier's Weekly*, and other nineteenth-century periodicals as well as on a range of decorative objects in middle-class American homes. Throughout the country, her admirers hung Gibson Girl prints on their walls and placed published collections of Gibson's work on their parlor tables. Her image appeared on porcelain plates, silver spoons, chair backs, pillow covers, and wallpaper. Through the popular nineteenth-century wood-burning craft of pyrography, her likeness could also be applied at home to an even wider variety of store-bought items, including wood and leather tabletops, glove boxes, umbrella stands, and other home

furnishings.[4] She influenced clothing fashions and hairstyles and was emulated by young women from as far afield as "New York and Boston, Grand Rapids and Sioux City."[5] Gibson's drawings were frequently reenacted as *tableaux vivants* at parties, charity bazaars, and church events. Songs such as "Why Do They Call Me a Gibson Girl?" were written in her honor, and she inspired plays, dances, and even a movie.

The Gibson Girl was a gentle rebel. She mirrored both the realities of girls' unprecedented freedoms and the anxieties that accompanied them. From 1890 until about 1910 Gibson gave his girl a range of new behaviors, and specific details of her features and clothing varied slightly from image to image. Yet she remained an essentially recognizable figure. While the circumstances in which she was depicted changed, her bodily presence did not. She was always tall and arranged her hair in a soft, upswept style. She wore the latest fashions, and whether dressed in a ball gown or the more typical stiff shirtwaist and long flowing skirt, she had an impossibly tiny waist.[6] She routinely engaged in newly acceptable activities for women: she played golf and croquet, rode a bicycle, and drove a motor car. She was never in quiet repose, like the women in Dewing's paintings, nor was she engaged in the introspective contemplation modeled by Eakins's subjects. In fact, she was rarely alone, and when she was she prepared for the moment she would be seen, looking in a mirror or adjusting her hair or clothing (fig. 28). Despite her independence, she was constantly aware of being looked at—both by figures who accompanied her in Gibson's drawings and by the viewer. She flirted. She was charming, but the cool, appraising cast of her eyes could border on haughty. She moved in the highest circles of society and attracted attention wherever she went. She could appear cool and detached, but there was typically something mischievous in her expression. She was often presented with a blend of admiration and satire. Occasionally she was pictured with other Gibson Girls, or as the most confident, elegant figure among a group of women (fig. 29). Most often, she appeared in the company of men, and she was frequently paired with a tall, clean-shaven, strong-jawed type who came to be known as the Gibson Man.[7]

The Gibson Girl modeled a new type of womanhood

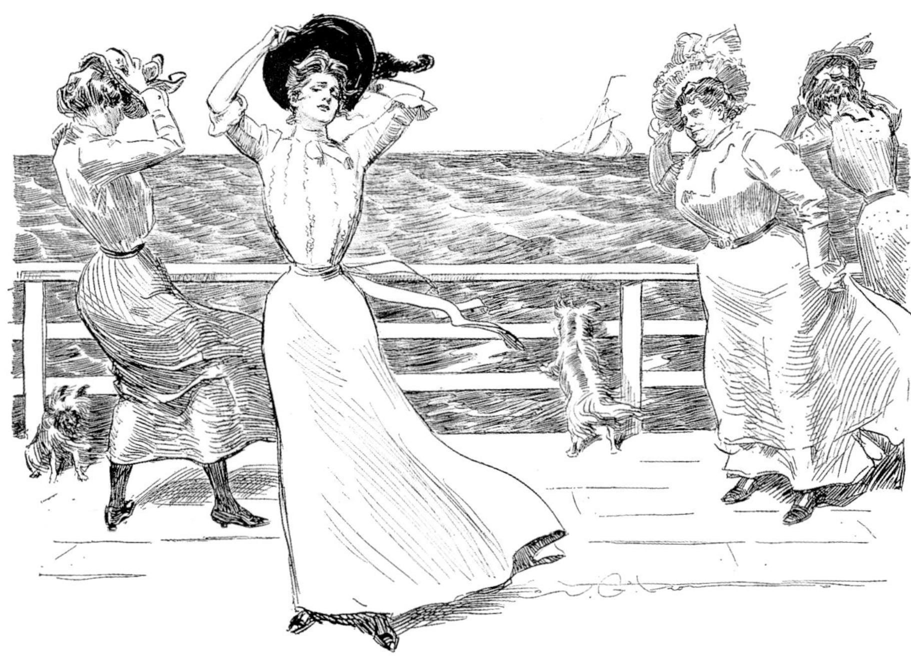

in the 1890s, quite unlike the painted and printed images of the passive women in dimly lit interiors that had come before her. In contrast to those images, the Gibson Girl was energetic and active, young, and vivacious. She made herself attractive and was interested in relationships with men, but she also exhibited new ambitions and interests outside the home. Somewhere in her early twenties, she was old enough to be courted but decidedly not married. She was a perfect creature of her moment, taking shape at a time when traditional gender relations and roles for women were undergoing radical change. Like many actual young women at the turn of the century, she struggled to find a place among competing models of American womanhood, and this struggle often centered on the question of marriage. Would she become a proper married "lady" like her mother, deferring to men and remaining quietly in the home as a virtuous moral guardian for her family? Or would she grow up to be a New Woman who went to high school and college, entered professions outside the home, fought for social equality with men, and often chose not to marry or have children? Gibson presented her enjoying many of the freedoms available to women, yet he also repeatedly placed her in romantic situations suggesting that she would ultimately marry. He never showed her going off to college, becoming involved in political or social

reform, or pursuing a career. Whatever else about the Gibson Girl was unpredictable, her interest in romance remained a constant.

The Gibson Girl's youth is significant. She was not a woman but a *girl*, as understood by late nineteenth-century culture. In the nineteenth century, girlhood—which included genteel, unmarried young women under 25 years of age—was a new and special category. Jane Hunter's recent study of the independent identities and social groups formed by nineteenth-century high school girls suggests that it was among "New Girls" rather than New Women that the first significant challenges to traditional women's roles were made. Hunter argues that the American Girl was granted a special status free from adult work and responsibilities and remained exempt—at least for a time—from the more restrictive expectations of gentility and ladyhood. Because it was generally assumed that girls would ultimately take up a traditional lady's role and responsibilities, girlhood was a time of unique freedoms, and girls were able to sidestep contemporary debate about the proper place for women in society.[8]

At the turn of the century, the Gibson Girl was the new American Girl as Hunter describes her. Like the growing number of girls who were attending school and developing relationships and interests outside the home

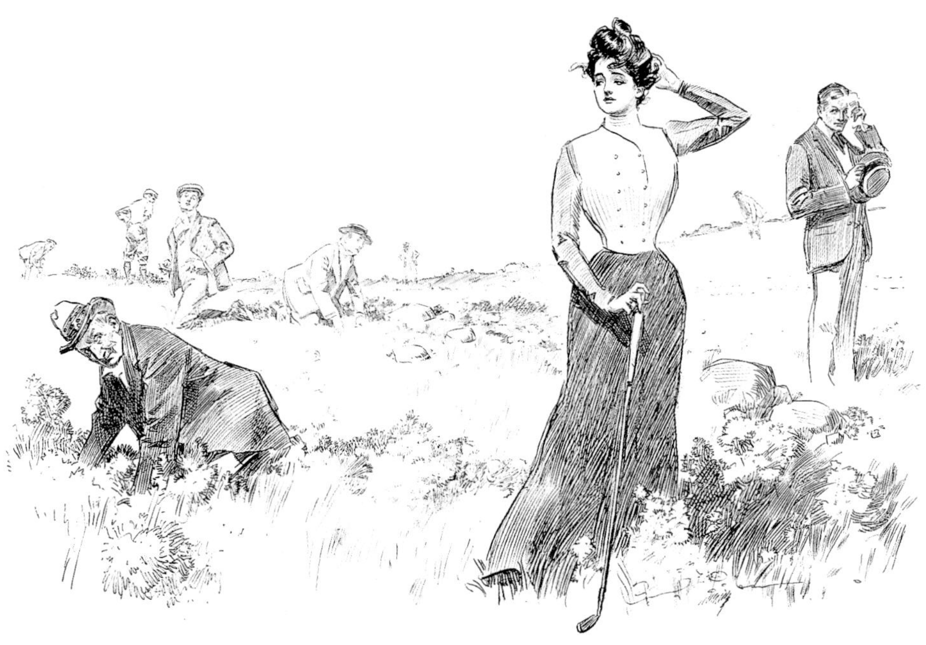

before establishing households of their own, the Gibson Girl explored an unprecedented period of independence between childhood and the assumption of conventional adult responsibilities. She had not yet decided which path to take. She was young and unmarried, beyond puberty but still innocent and girlish. She was the peer and equal of young men, and she was active both within and outside the home. She rejected the restrictive ideals of an older generation and moved significantly beyond the traditional domestic world associated with women, yet she remained interested in becoming a wife and mother.

The Gibson Girl's relationships with men are a constant focus in Gibson's drawings. *Advice to Caddies*, which Gibson published in 1900, is a typical image of the Gibson Girl's relations with the opposite sex (fig. 30). Her involvement in sports here is highlighted not as a primarily athletic activity but as a respectable opportunity for her to socialize—unchaperoned—with young men. She stands imperiously in the foreground, touching her hair coyly with one hand while idly holding a golf club in the other. Her skirt and tendrils of her hair blow gently in the breeze as she looks off into the distance with a patient—if somewhat bored—expression. She is surrounded by a group of distracted men who search vainly for golf balls, their efforts frustrated by their inability to

pay attention to anything other than the beautiful and seductive Gibson Girl in the foreground. The drawing's subtitle—"You will save time by keeping your eye on the ball, not the player"—is comic but also hints at deeper anxieties about the Gibson Girl's allure. While she is clearly the object of the male gaze in this image, she controls it. The young man standing behind her seems speechless in her presence; the most he can do is mop the sweat from his brow and sneak a glance in her direction. The Gibson Girl may be playing the modern sport of golf and wearing new, less confining clothing, but she is also a stunning beauty whose charms overpower men. She has brought the men around her—literally, in many cases—to their knees.

Many of Gibson's drawings clearly expressed anxiety about the power and independence of the American Girl and about the fact that her future was undecided. What seems to soften her threat is the implication that she would ultimately marry.[9] By focusing on courtship and relationships between the Gibson Girl and the men around her, Gibson linked the uncertain—and potentially dangerous—figure of the American Girl to a more familiar—and less threatening—pattern of life for women. For young women who remained single, he forecast a gloomy future.[10] In *The Spinster's Revery* (fig. 31), a worn old woman sits slumped in a chair,

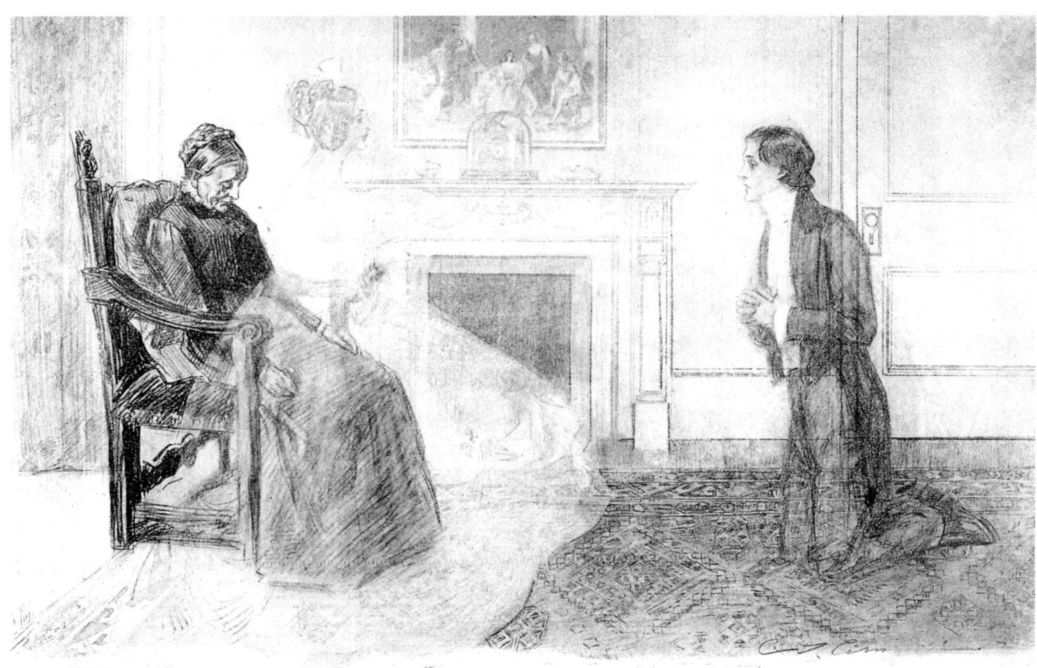

dreaming that she is again young and being wooed by a suitor. Now alone in her old age, the shriveled spinster has nothing but this memory of her youth, when she coolly turned down the young man who wanted to marry her. In *People Who* Will *Have Their Own Way: The Girl Who Refused Us* (fig. 32) Gibson graphically outlines the consequences for his independent girls if they refuse marriage. The sequence of images begins with the familiar Gibson Girl, beautiful and aloof, her back to the viewer. In the next panel she is slightly older, her face is lined, and she has become more concerned with whomever may be watching. She is turned to the side and gazes over her shoulder with a smile. In the third panel she is older still, with a thinner face and frame and more heavily lined skin. She is now turned almost entirely toward the viewer but wears a smaller, less coquettish smile on her face. By the final panel she is thin, worn, wrinkled, and holds a lorgnette in one hand as she looks directly out at the viewer with a pursed expression on her deeply shadowed face. She has physically withered, her punishment for not marrying.

In case there is any confusion about what the spinster and the "girl who refused us" have given up, the viewer need only look to drawings like *After Fifteen Years, When She Refused Him He Vowed He Would Never Marry*, in which a fashionably dressed woman—no longer a fresh-faced Gibson Girl—is confronted by a former suitor, who is now happily married and the father of the five young children who accompany him (fig. 33). Perhaps she too is now married; the evidence suggests otherwise. She is alone, and as he tips his hat and smiles in her direction she returns his gaze with a pinched face, now heavier than it once was, and clasps a book tightly in her hands. She and her fellow spinsters are Gibson Girls who have failed their potential. They have lost not only their youth but also the Gibson Girl's characteristic beauty, spirit, and appeal. Unlike their fragile lady predecessors, they do not succumb to nervous illnesses, but they lose their beauty and female fulfillment.

The anxiety underlying Gibson's investment in marriage became more pronounced the farther the Gibson Girl strayed from the civilizing environment of the home. Particularly when surrounded by elements such as wind and water, the threat she posed intensified. In such instances, Gibson fashioned her as an American femme fatale, a popular female type at the turn of the century. Femmes fatales embody danger. Irresistibly attractive, they lure men only to destroy them. In *Not the Sea Serpent, but Far More Dangerous*, a smiling Gibson Girl swims in the ocean, a disembodied head visible above the water (fig. 34). Like a sea serpent, she is at home in

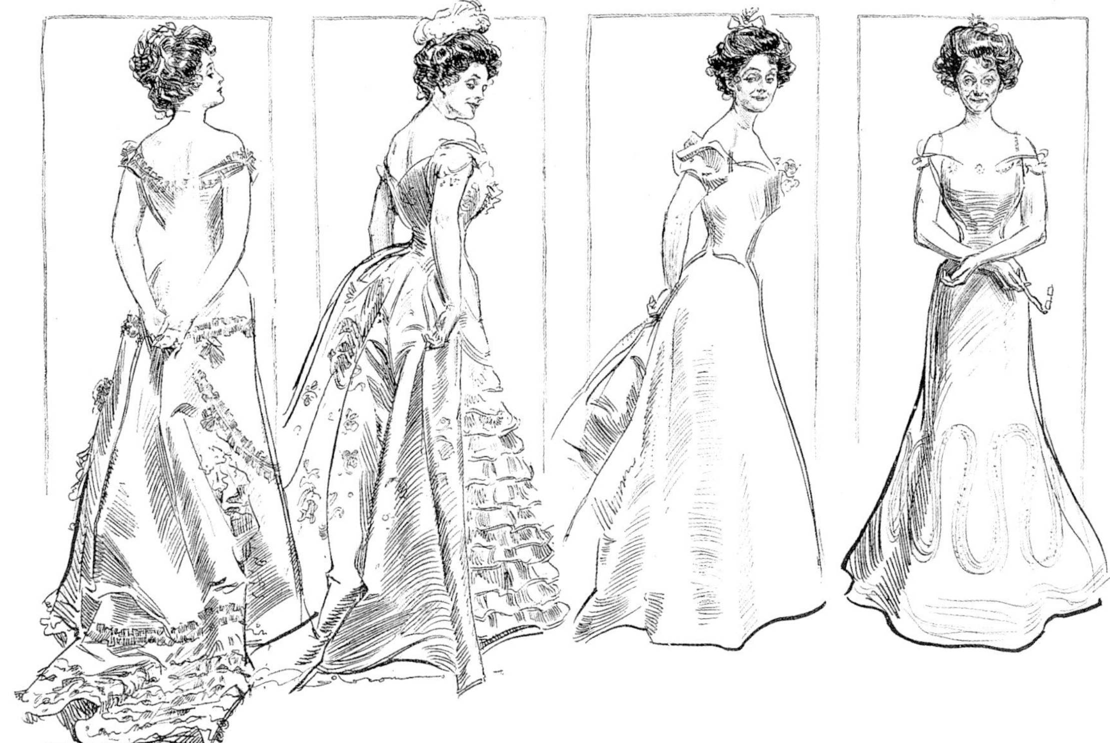

FIG. 32 [*right*]
Charles Dana Gibson,
*People Who Will Have
Their Own Way: The Girl
Who Refused Us*, 1899.

FIG. 33 [*below*]
Charles Dana Gibson,
*After Fifteen Years, When She
Refused Him He Vowed He
Would Never Marry*, 1903.

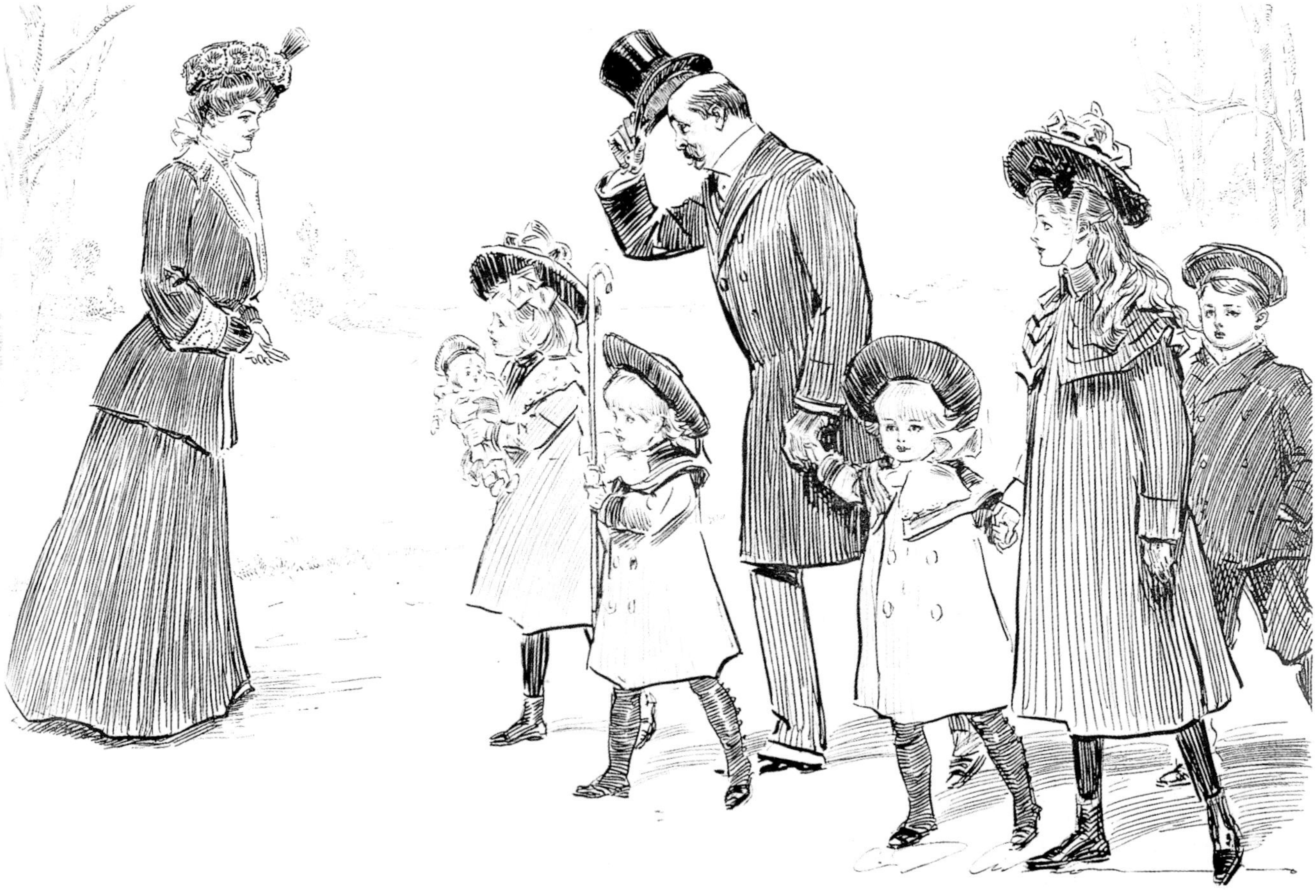

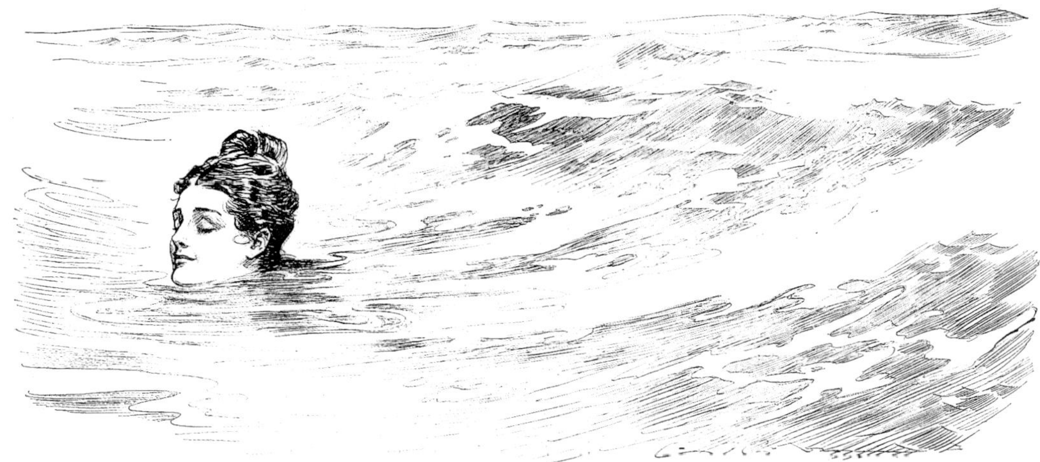

the powerful waves, daring her male to enter the water with her. She appears relaxed; her eyes are closed, and she smiles sweetly. She is completely at home in the water and in control of her situation. Perhaps more to the point, she is beautiful. It is her beauty, as well as the innocence of her expression, that make her such a threat. She seems docile and inviting, but like a sea serpent she is poised to destroy those who might join her for a swim.

It is this combination of threat and attraction that defines the femme fatale. She appears submissive and feminine, yet she is powerful and manipulative. In European femme fatale imagery, she often preys on and destroys men.[11] Gibson's femmes fatales were less violent figures, but even in their softened state they belonged to the genre.[12] Gibson drew very few femmes fatales, but those he completed revealed an amplified nervousness about the potential consequences of women's new freedoms. The anxiety expressed in these images was present to one degree or another in all of Gibson's drawings. For many Americans at the turn of the century, the New Girl was considered just as threatening a figure as the femme fatale. She could enact the ideal of what a virtuous woman was supposed to be, or she could embody all that was disquieting about the independent and sexually free New Woman. According to historian Jean V. Matthews, one reason for the restrictive codes of ladydom was the assumption that relations between men and women—especially the younger ones—"were potentially sexual in nature and had to be hedged about

with external and internalized prohibitions to protect the purity—and thus marriageability—of young women."[13] Donald Mrozek has made a similar argument, demonstrating that in the nineteenth century it was feared that women were by nature "excessively sexual" beings: "The 'weakness' of the weaker sex did not mean that [women] could not harm men; it meant rather that they were morally weak and in a sense out of control."[14] Mrozek, like Matthews, suggests that the ideal of "ladylike" behavior was invoked as a means of keeping this sexual threat in check.[15]

Gibson contained the threat New Girls posed by implicitly framing them in a reassuring courtship narrative. In his typical boy-girl flirtation, the Gibson Man had to struggle to attain the woman of his dreams, but in the end, he prevailed. The thrill of the chase that Gibson drawings dramatize was a large part of their appeal—particularly for turn-of-the-century men. One male contemporary noted in 1897, "We perceive that there is something to conquer. For the girl whom the artist gives us is not a ready prey to sentiment and does not yield very easily.... Love must stalk his game; though confident of success in the end, he is strategic in his approaches."[16] The fact that the Gibson Man ultimately had the upper hand was for contemporary viewers "a true testament" to the Gibson Girl's "purity of heart and healthy soundness of nature."[17] In other words, by falling in love and choosing to marry, the Gibson Girl proved that she was a "pure" and "natural"

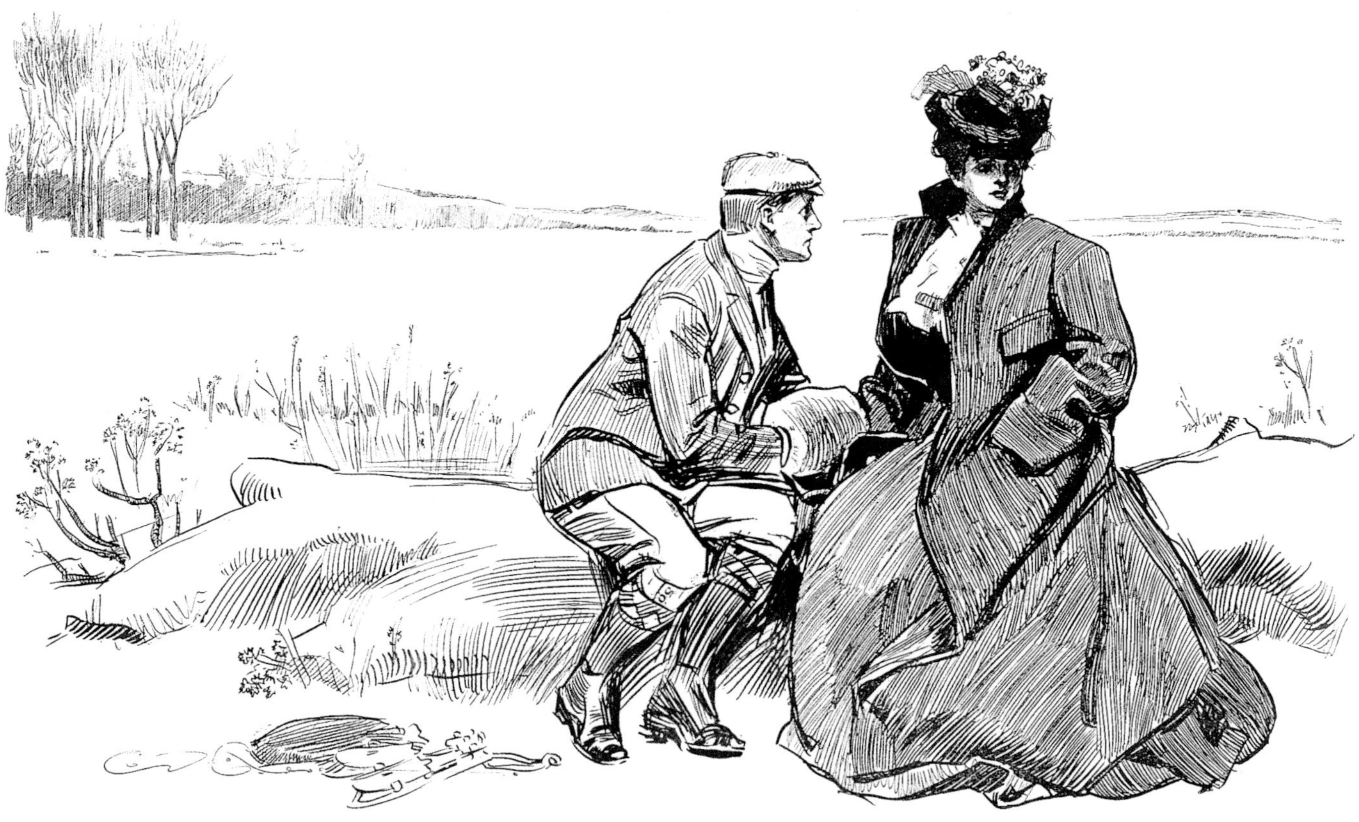

FIG. 35 Charles Dana Gibson, *Melting*, 1900.

woman, not corrupted by the social changes that were leading women to pursue professions outside the home and to postpone—or refuse—marriage. Her eventual submission to the Gibson Man reassured male viewers that their bewildering attraction to the Gibson Girl need not trouble them for long; it would be controlled once she assumed her role as wife and mother.

To woo the Gibson Girl was to bring an uncontainable and potentially threatening power under control. In *Melting*, a couple sits outdoors in a wintry landscape, a pair of ice skates cast off near their feet (fig. 35). The Gibson Girl turns away from the young man at her side and gazes off almost expressionlessly into the distance. She is bundled in a heavy coat with one hand in her pocket, and she appears aloof and detached. Then we notice that her other hand shares a muff with the hand of the young man beside her. He is making progress, and her icy reserve is melting. In *The Turning of the Tide*, the young man's victory is even more complete (fig. 36). This time the Gibson Girl is identified not with ice but

with another natural element: the ocean in which the couple sits. They are kissing, apparently so absorbed in each other that they are unaware of the water now surrounding them. Curiously the Gibson Girl, who appears to actually be closest to the shore, seems to be more deeply submerged in the water than her lover, and almost to be a part of it. Were the water to continue its rise she might become Gibson's femme fatale figure and destroy her man. But the tide is turning, as the drawing's caption reminds us, and we see now that she wears an engagement ring on her left hand—a detail Gibson has left conspicuously visible along with the couple's clasped hands. Their engagement has turned the tide in the Gibson Man's favor, and he is gaining ground. The Gibson Girl's submission will follow.

Gibson often employed humor to soften the threat posed by his independent women, particularly when he depicted them in narratives other than courtship. In *Summer Sports*, his three playful young girls relax on a windy hillside (fig. 37). They appear to be flying kites,

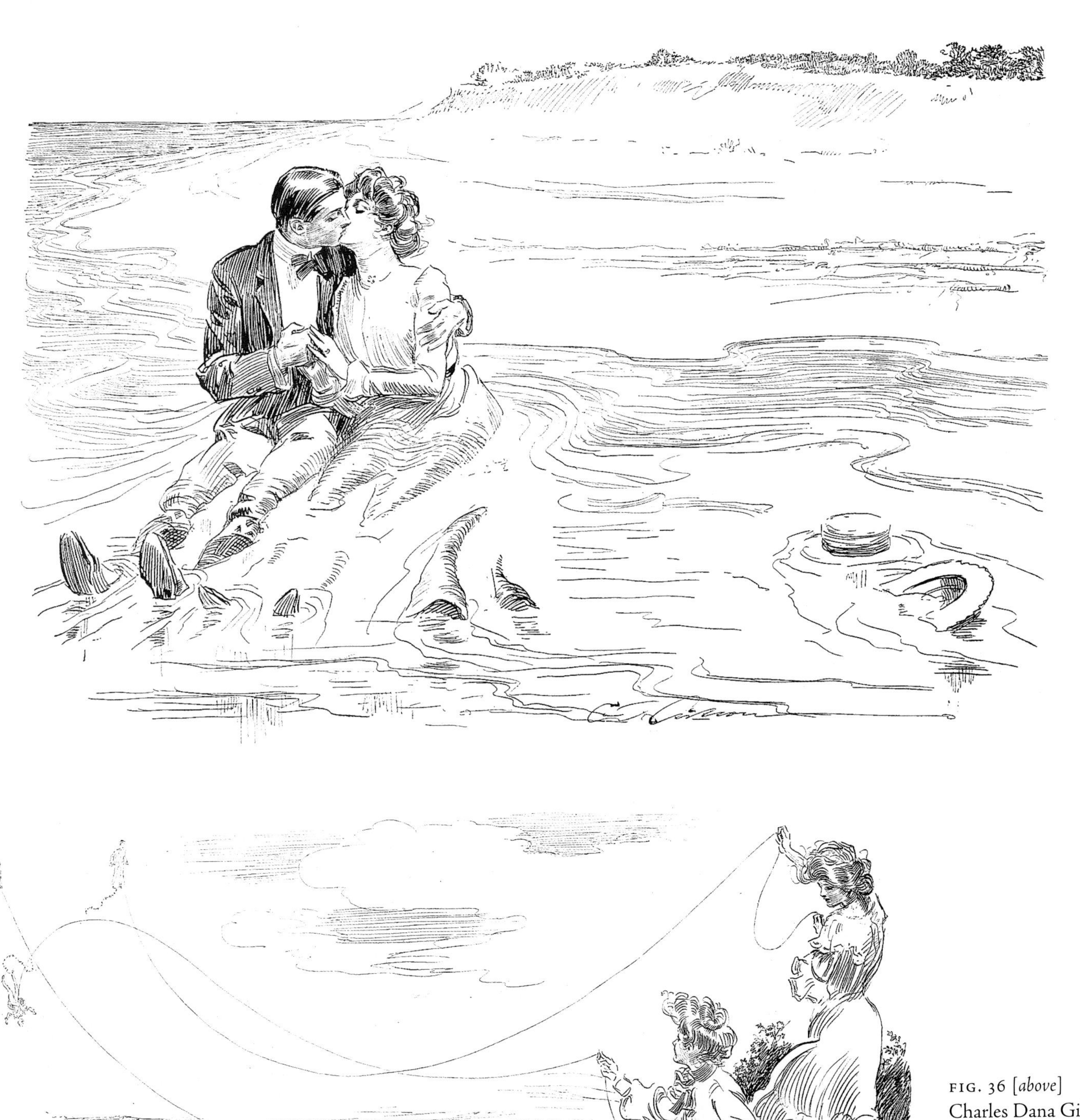

FIG. 36 [*above*]
Charles Dana Gibson,
The Turning of the Tide,
1901.

FIG. 37 [*left*]
Charles Dana Gibson,
Summer Sports, 1904.

but after looking more closely we see men at the end of their kite strings—small men, who in comparison to the robust young women appear as lifeless and powerless as dolls. One of them dangles upside down, while another has just lost his hat. Here it is the women who are pulling the strings, and we have no clear indication of when—or if—they will decide to reel in the men. Clearly, when marriage—and the domestication of the Gibson Girl that it implies—is uncertain, the threat to men becomes real. These women are no longer dangerous and desirable femmes fatales but rather monstrous puppeteers, able to control the men on their kite strings at a whim. Yet their behavior is so improbable as to provoke laughter. In the end, the shifting of power relations in this image is exposed as nothing but an anxious fantasy, exaggerated to the point of comedy.

The women in *The Turning of the Tide* and *Summer Sports* are on opposite sides of the line carefully walked by most of the Gibson Girl drawings—and many actual young women—at the turn of the century. Would they submit to men or control their own destiny? Or would they try to find a balance between traditional duties and relationships and their new independence? As Caroline Ticknor's story "The Steel-Engraving Lady and the Gibson Girl" suggests, these questions were a frequent topic of commentary in turn-of-the-century periodicals.[18] The strongest challenger to the prevailing lady ideal was less the Gibson Girl than the New Woman, a figure just coming into focus in the 1890s when the Gibson Girl first appeared. By the turn of the century, when Ticknor's story was published, the New Woman was more clearly defined, and Ticknor's Gibson Girl incorporates some of the New Woman's characteristics. She had been to college and was active outside the home, not as a socialite but as a professional and a reformer. Though she had a boyfriend, romantic relationships were not her first priority.

The historian Carroll Smith-Rosenberg has identified two generations of New Women. The first generation attended women's colleges in the 1870s and 1880s and participated in activities and occupations outside the home. But they also generally adhered to traditional ideals of family life and accepted genteel codes of conduct. The second generation of New

Women—contemporaries of the Gibson Girl—were educated in the 1890s and came into their own in the years immediately before and after World War I. This second generation was more radical than the first; these women often had careers, remained unmarried, and were activists for causes such as women's suffrage that scandalized many Americans at the time.[19] The Gibson Girl is sometimes characterized today as a New Woman, and in Ticknor's story she takes on many of these qualities, but in fact she had more in common with Smith-Rosenberg's first generation of New Women than with the more radical second generation who appeared in visual culture a bit later.[20] By the standards of her time, the Gibson Girl was a new type—and certainly presented a clear departure from the restrictions placed on the lady—yet she bore little resemblance to the popular image of the New Woman whom Ticknor's Gibson Girl resembles. In the 1890s the "mannish," radical type represented by second-generation New Women was an exaggerated, grotesque figure in popular cartoons, novels, and magazine and newspaper articles. She was dangerous not because of her sexual attractiveness to men, but rather because she was an "unsexed, terrifying, violent Amazon ready to overturn the world."[21]

The Gibson Girl was always an ambiguous figure, and her creator seemed by turns to love her, fear her, and wish to contain her and the changes she represented.[22] Gibson never allowed his girls to become political activists. Indeed, he was not sympathetic to organized feminism, and he feared that women's involvement in politics would make them coarser and more masculine. Gibson Girls were independent, but they were rarely "mannish."[23] John Ames Mitchell, the founder and editor of *Life*, explained that one of the reasons he first accepted Gibson's drawings was that the Gibson Girl was a lady.[24] It would have been more accurate to say that the Gibson Girl would become a lady. In her life as a popular drawing she remained an American Girl, a category that was a fashionable female ideal all its own and continued to be illustrated well into the twentieth century by artists such as Harrison Fisher and Howard Chandler Christy.

Ticknor's elision of the relatively moderate Gibson

Girl and the more radical New Woman suggests that for many viewers the anxiety produced by any disruption of traditional gender roles ignored such fine distinctions. At a time when the roles and responsibilities of actual women were undergoing radical change many Americans sought continuity and reassurance in visual representations of female types.[25] Both Gibson's drawings of spirited New Girls and the intellectual, passive ladies painted by artists such as Dewing, Alexander, and Tarbell respond to the unease caused by shifting gender roles in the late nineteenth century. While paintings of the Woman at Home celebrate and reinforce the confining ideal of ladydom, the assurance that the Gibson Girl would become a wife and mother kept the threat posed by her freedom and independence in check. It was when Gibson focused on subjects that strayed farthest from the reassuring Gibson Girl model—such as spinsters, femmes fatales, and children—that his deep ambivalence about shifting gender roles became most clear.

Gibson's drawings of the "little American Girl" are particularly telling. Younger than the flirtatious Gibson Girl, the little American Girl had a more ambiguous future. Even in her youth she had an unsettling power over the opposite sex. She could grow up to become a lady, or she could choose an altogether different path. In *The Nursery* we see her sitting in a chair with a doll in her lap, holding the ends of a rope that is attached—like reins—to a young boy crouching before her on his hands and knees (fig. 38). While the boy stares at the ground, oblivious to the viewer, the young girl looks out with a coy half smile on her face—an expression not unlike that of many Gibson Girls. Because she remains too young to be truly dangerous, the little American Girl has a power over the boy that her older sister would never have been allowed. *The Nursery* calls to mind *Summer Sports*, and one might imagine this little American Girl eventually sitting among her older sisters, confidently holding the kite strings while powerless men float in the distance like toys. While the women in *Summer Sports* are older, their preposterous situation prevents the danger they pose from ever being realized. In *The Nursery*, the little American Girl's youth likewise undermines her threatening behavior, yet the implications of

the image remain terrifying. The girl's actions call attention to the unsettling potential of all little American girls in a time of expanding possibilities for women.

In Gibson's most popular drawings, he assured viewers that the threats posed by new opportunities for women could be contained. The Gibson Girl's happy march toward the altar and motherhood rarely admitted uncertainty about the future. Yet in images like *The Nursery* Gibson gave voice to a question that haunted many Americans at the turn of the twentieth century: what might the future of American womanhood be? With the drawing *Yes or No* (fig. 39), which appeared in *Collier's Weekly* in 1906, Gibson approached an answer. In this instance we see a young woman who bears only a faint resemblance to the Gibson Girl, and who seems ready to move beyond that role entirely. She is seated at a table writing a letter—presumably to a suitor—and has completed only one line, which appears to read "Dear Tom." She has paused for a moment and looks up with a thoughtful expression on her face. She doesn't flirt or smile. In fact, she doesn't seem to see the viewer at all; she gazes seriously at some unfixed point in the distance. She is young and attractive, but she does not wear the usual sleek and fashionable clothing of the Gibson Girl, and her hair is arranged in a looser, less formal style. She is not in public, on display before all the world; instead, we find her in a quiet moment, contemplating her future. As the title suggests, she must answer Tom "yes or no." In this moment, she must decide which life to choose. This Gibson Girl was on the verge of being a New Woman, one with the freedom to determine her own future. The choices she and other young women like her made would have serious implications for the traditional Victorian social order.

In *Yes or No* Gibson did not attempt to resolve the questions and uncertainties raised by increased freedoms for women. Instead, he presented a truly new girl who had the power to decide her own future. Such girls were rare in Gibson's work. The playful Gibson Girl, with her certain future in the arms of the Gibson Man, was far more popular. In contrast with this young woman—and the many actual young women like her—visual types such as the Gibson Girl, the neurasthenic, or the Woman at Home painted by artists like

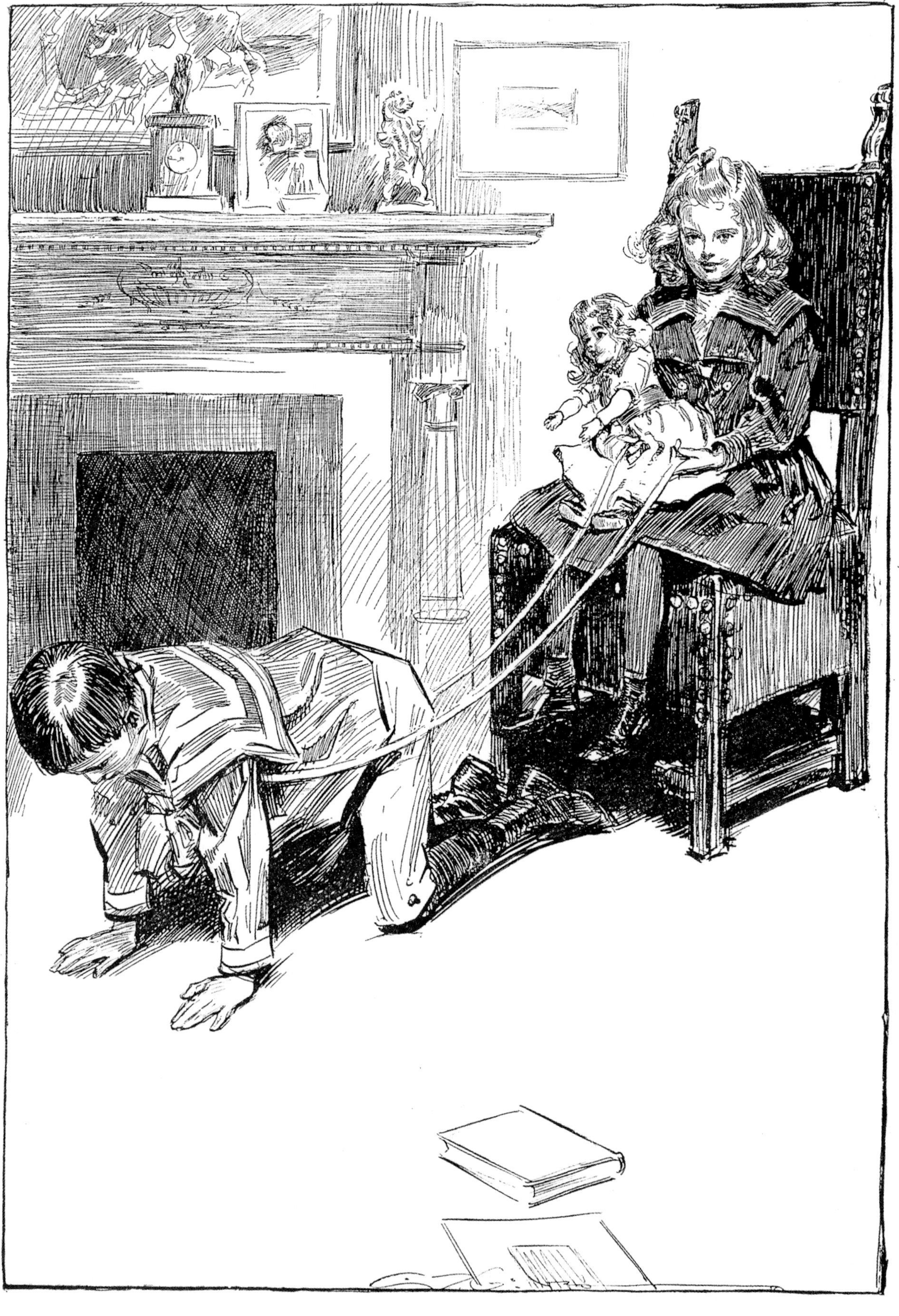

Dewing and Tarbell offered the fantasy many turn-of-the-century viewers sought. The Gibson Girl had more freedom and independence than the aestheticized women painted in luxurious interiors, yet she was not a deeply threatening reformer. As a fairly ambivalent figure who reflected and filtered behaviors and activities engaged in by turn-of-the-century young women, Gibson's American Girl modeled a balance of traditional roles and new opportunities—but she would ultimately fall in love. In the courtship and marriage of the Gibson Girl the threats of New Womanhood were averted; New Girls became New Ladies.

Notes

I would like to thank Claire Perry, Bernard Barryte, Jeanie Lawrence, and, especially, Wanda Corn, without whom this essay would never have come to be.

1. Caroline Ticknor, "The Steel-Engraving Lady and the Gibson Girl," *The Atlantic Monthly* (July 1901): 105–8. Ticknor was a frequent contributor to *The Atlantic Monthly*.

2. Lois Banner, who draws the term "steel-engraving lady" from Ticknor's story, devotes a chapter to discussing this nineteenth-century ideal. See "The Ideal Woman: The Steel-Engraving Lady," in Lois W. Banner, *American Beauty: A Social History, Through Two Centuries, of the American Idea, Ideal, and Image of the Beautiful Woman* (New York: Alfred A. Knopf, 1983), 45–65.

3. It was in this period that the first large-scale publishing operations emerged, and circulation dramatically increased. In 1865 there were 700 magazines with a total circulation of four million, and in 1905 those numbers had jumped to 6,000 titles with a total of sixty-four million subscribers, averaging four magazine subscriptions per household. See Carolyn Kitch, *The Girl on the Magazine Cover: The Origins of Visual Stereotypes in American Mass Media* (Chapel Hill: University of North Carolina Press, 2001), 4. In addition to supplying an interesting analysis of female visual types, Kitch provides a useful history of the development of American magazines.

4. For discussion of Gibson Girl–inspired popular culture, see Richard Harding Davis, "Charles Dana Gibson's Pictures: The Origins of a Type of the American Girl," *Monthly Illustrator* 3 (January 3, 1895): 6; Henry C. Pitz, "Charles Dana Gibson: Creator of a Mode," *American Artist* 20 (December 1956): 50–55; Agnes Rogers, "The Undimmed Appeal of the Gibson Girl," *American Heritage* 9 (December 1957): 97; and Robert Koch, "Gibson Girl Revisited," *Art in America* 53 (1965): 70–71. The "re-domestication" suggested by the appearance of the Gibson Girl on objects for the home raises interesting issues but has not been well documented.

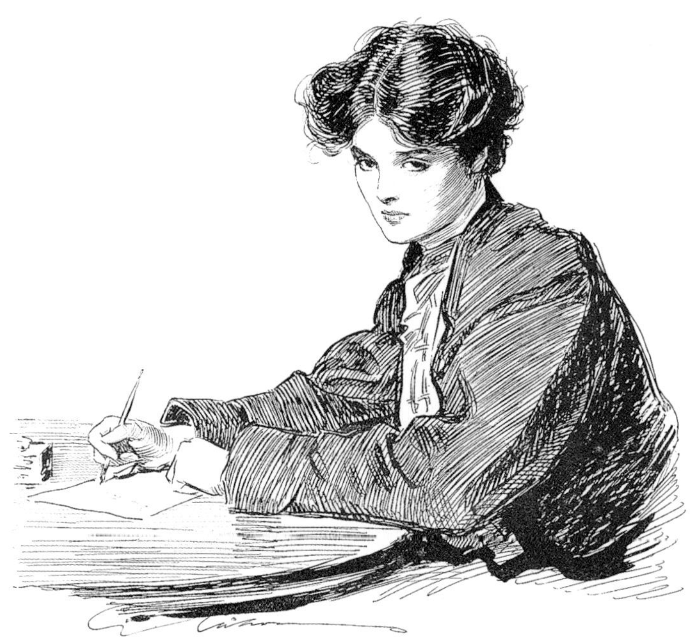

FIG. 39 Charles Dana Gibson, *Yes or No*, 1906.

Pitz's article—which includes no footnotes, illustrations, or references to manufacturers or designers—mentions numerous examples of popular objects based on the Gibson Girl motif and has been widely cited by later scholars. Koch provides patent dates and manufacturers for many of the examples he includes but illustrates only one item—a dresser set—directly based on the Gibson Girl. His other examples are more generalized, art nouveau designs, including women and floral patterns, which he suggests are related to Gibson Girl imagery.

5. Davis, 6.

6. My thanks to Ellen Wiley Todd for sharing with me the transcript of a talk she gave at the Clark Institute in February 2003: "Making a Waist: Workers, Wearers, and Fashion's Image before the 1911 Triangle Fire," drawn from her current book project, *The "Infamous Blaze": Visual Imagery, Cultural Memory, and the Triangle Shirtwaist Fire*. Todd explores the shirtwaist as a "material embodiment of and a symbolic repository for debates on class, gender, and women's changing occupational and public roles at the turn of the century." Her analysis will significantly enrich our understanding of the new fashions worn by the Gibson Girl. Clothing was a focus for Gibson; he remarked to an interviewer in 1901 that wearing the appropriate clothing was one of the defining characteristics of the Gibson Girl: "It is instinctively born in an American girl to wear the proper thing at the proper time. Their

FIG. 38 [*facing*] Charles Dana Gibson, *The Nursery*, 1899.

taste is never at fault, and they are consequently the best-groomed women in any international gathering." (See Francis Arnold Collins, "The 'Father' of the American Girl: Mr. Charles Dana Gibson," *London Magazine* 7 [November 1901]: 343.) It is worth noting that the Gibson Girl's clothing was not particularly comfortable. While the Gibson Girl look lacked bustles and draping and was without many of the fussy details of earlier styles, the waist remained tightly cinched, the skirt was excessively long and tight around the hips, and the full sleeves of the Gibson Girl's trademark shirtwaist partially immobilized her arms. The celebrated "reform corset" worn by the Gibson Girl (which used suspenders to flatten the abdomen, thereby causing less interference with breathing) was an improvement but continued to inhibit fully free movement. See Kathryn Weibel, "Images of Fashionable Women," in *Mirror Mirror: Images of Women Reflected in Popular Culture* (Garden City, NY: Anchor Books, 1977), 175–222.

7. See Banner, and Rogers, 97.

8. The most comprehensive discussion of the development of the American Girl is offered by Jane H. Hunter, *How Young Ladies Became Girls: The Victorian Origins of American Girlhood* (New Haven: Yale University Press, 2002). See also Claudia Nelson and Lynn Valone, eds., *The Girl's Own: Cultural Histories of the Anglo-American Girl, 1830–1915* (Athens: University of Georgia Press, 1994).

9. Even when Gibson's drawings addressed broader topics such as wealth, self-deception, and social climbing, he typically explored these issues in the context of interactions between men and women. Interestingly, Chris Willis has observed that the figure in British popular fiction of the late 1890s (whom she calls the "commercialized New Woman") typically appeared in stories "written by men—perhaps attempting to defuse the threat of the New Woman by emphasizing her youth, sexual attractiveness, and the supposed folly of her desire for independence." These women were "attractive, independent, highly intelligent young women entering a range of professions before (almost invariably) falling in love" and assuming a wifely role. It seems that something similar is operating in Gibson's work. See Willis, "'Heaven Defend Me from Political or Highly-Educated Women!': Packaging the New Woman for Mass Consumption," in *The New Woman in Fact and Fiction*, ed. Angelique Richardson and Chris Willis (Hampshire, Eng.: Palgrave Macmillan, Ltd., 2001), 53–65.

10. In 1895 Richard Harding Davis wrote "with all of his evident admiration for the American girl, Gibson is somewhat inconsistent. For he is constantly placing her in positions that make us fear she is a cynical and worldly-wise young person, and of a fickleness that belies her looks." As a result of this tendency, the artist's friends were often asked if Gibson was "a disappointed lover himself, and in consequence a little morbid and a good deal of a cynic" (Davis, 6).

11. For a discussion of femme fatale imagery in turn-of-the-century art, see Bram Dijkstra, *Idols of Perversity: Fantasies of Feminine Evil in Fin-de-Siècle Culture* (New York: Oxford University Press, 1986). Although Djikstra focuses on European examples, he includes a discussion of Gibson's drawing *In the Swim: Dedicated to Extravagant Women*, 1900. See also Martha Kingsbury, "The Femme Fatale and Her Sisters," *Art News Annual* 38 (1972): 191–95. Kingsbury discusses Gibson's *A Northeaster*, 1900 (fig. 29).

12. Rebecca Stott's definition of the femme fatale is useful, though she focuses on the type as a literary figure. See Stott, *The Fabrication of the Late-Victorian Femme Fatale* (London: Macmillan Press, 1992).

13. Jean V. Matthews, *The Rise of the New Woman: The Woman's Movement in America, 1875–1930* (Chicago: Uvan R. Dee, 2003), 10. Susan Wolstenholme has likewise suggested that young women posed a particular threat. The Gibson Girl's youth (and, by implication, virginal purity) rendered her immune to the sexual drive she compelled in men, and she was therefore especially dangerous. Wolstenholme, "Edith Wharton's Gibson Girl: The Virgin, the Undine, and the Dynamo," *American Literary Realism* 18 (1985): 92–107. On the Gibson Girl as a sexualized figure see also Martha Banta, *Imaging American Women: Idea and Ideals in Cultural History* (New York: Columbia University Press, 1987), 216, and Koch, 70. Koch, whose brief article (published in 1965) is frequently cited by more recent scholars, likely influenced many subsequent readings of the Gibson Girl with his statement "The Gibson Girl has a touch of Venus, a flavor of the French music-hall, and the character of the emancipated woman. Well dressed in the latest fashion, often innocently in love, she soon became the first all American pin-up girl." Interestingly, Agnes Rogers, in her characterization of the Gibson Girl published eight years earlier (1957), suggested that the Gibson Girl was far less sexualized than contemporary images of women: "She was femininity incarnate, without being (in today's terms) sexy. And nowadays, when sex is portrayed in such blatant detail, it is refreshing to be given the promise of future raptures rather than the play-by-play accounts of bedroom romps in current novels," 80. It is possible that the gender of these authors influenced their readings of the Gibson Girl.

14. Donald J. Mrozek, "The 'Amazon' and the American 'Lady': Sexual Fears of Women as Athletes," in *From Fair Sex to Feminism: Sport and the Socialization of Women in the Industrial and Post-Industrial Eras*, ed. J. A. Mangan and Roberta J. Park (London: Frank Cass and Co., 1987), 283. Of course, not all men were threatened by new freedoms for women. Michael Kimmel has identified three distinctive categories of response to turn-of-the-century feminism. See Kimmel, "Men's Responses to Feminism at the Turn of the Century," *Gender and Society* 1 (September 1987): 261–83.

15. The Gibson Girl's impossibly thin waist may also have signified an anxious interest in self-control. Peter Stearns has identified the Gibson Girl's slender figure as a marker of a new emphasis on thinness, which became characteristic of the ideal female body type in the 1890s. Stearns suggests that the new fash-

ion for weight loss promoted by the Gibson Girl was related to the fact that the ideal of motherhood was declining and women were increasingly able to explore their sexuality. "Dieting was a way, again, to express virtue and self-control even in a changing sexual climate." For further discussion of nineteenth-century changes in attitudes toward obesity, see Stearns's essay in the forthcoming collection *Cultures of the Abdomen*, ed. Christopher E. Forth and Ana Carden-Cayne, which will be published in November 2004. The book is described in Dinitia Smith, "Demonizing Fat in the War on Weight," *New York Times* (May 1, 2004). Lois Banner also briefly discusses the shift to a less voluptuous female type in the late nineteenth century. See Banner, 151–53.

16. Anthony Hope, "Mr. Charles Dana Gibson on Love and Life," *McClure's Magazine* 9 (August 1897): 870.

17. Ibid.

18. Several recent studies have considered literary representations of turn-of-the-century female types, but a comprehensive study of visual representations has yet to be completed. The Gibson Girl was the most pervasive and popular female type at the turn of the century. It seems that positive representations of the New Woman did not appear in the popular press until the 1920s. For general discussions of female ideals, see Banta, Banner, and Kitch. On the idealization of women in art, see Ann Uhry Abrams, "Frozen Goddess: The Image of Women in Nineteenth-Century Art," in *Woman's Being, Woman's Place: Female Identity and Vocation in American History*, ed. Mary Kelley (Boston: G. K. Hall, 1979), 93–108; and Bailey Van Hook, *Angels of Art: Women and Art in American Society, 1876–1914* (University Park: The Pennsylvania State University Press, 1996).

19. Carroll Smith-Rosenberg, "Bourgeois Discourse and the Progressive Era: An Introduction," in *Disorderly Conduct: Visions of Gender in Victorian America* (New York: Alfred A. Knopf, 1985), 176–77.

20. For discussion of the New Woman in visual culture, see Talia Schaffer, "'Nothing but Foolscap and Ink': Inventing the New Woman," in Richardson and Willis, 39–40. In the essay immediately following Schaffer's in the same volume, Chris Willis, writing about the New Woman figure in popular British fiction, makes a different argument. Willis argues that while the New Woman "was not always sympathetically portrayed in popular culture" and, like "her later counterpart the suffragette," was

"frequently caricatured as being ugly and unmarriageable," by the late 1890s "the image of the New Woman as a bicycling Amazon seems largely to have taken over from the image of her as an unattractive bluestocking." Willis sees the New Woman in popular fiction as "a commercialized version of the heroine of didactic New Woman fiction," yet she makes little of the fact that examples she cites such as the Girton Girl (named in honor of the first British women's college) are "invariably referred to as a 'girl' rather than a woman." It seems likely that several of the figures Willis describes might be better described as the type of new girls Hunter discusses. See Willis, 53–65.

21. Schaffer, "'Nothing but Foolscap and Ink,'" in Richardson and Willis, *The New Woman in Fact and Fiction*, 39–40.

22. Martha Patterson and Lynn Gordon have noted, respectively, ways in which the Gibson Girl transformed and contained threats posed by the new womanhood. See Patterson, "'Survival of the Best Fitted': Selling the American New Woman as Gibson Girl, 1895–1910," *ATQ* 9 (1992): 73–87; and Gordon, "The Gibson Girl Goes to College: Popular Culture and Women's Higher Education in the Progressive Era, 1890–1920," *American Quarterly* 39 (1987): 211–30. Along similar lines, scholars have begun to examine the ways in which transforming the New Woman into a stereotype might serve as a strategy of control. See the Introduction to Richardson and Willis, and Willis, in Richardson and Willis, 53–65.

23. See Banner, 157; and Ellen Wiley Todd, *The "New Woman" Revised: Painting and Gender Politics on Fourteenth Street* (Berkeley: University of California Press, 1993), 8. According to Todd, "Gibson mistrusted organized feminism, fearing it would make women too masculine. He deplored the extreme tactics of radical suffragists and, until his own wife served as a Democratic committeewoman, had reservations about women's political role."

24. Rogers, 80.

25. Most scholarship on gender and women's status at the turn of the twentieth century has been produced by historians. Art historian Ellen Wiley Todd's study *The "New" Woman Revised* demonstrates what can be gained by considering the visual images—both popular and fine art—informed by debates about separate spheres (and other aspects of women's advancement) at the turn of the century. Todd cites Boston School painters such as Edmund Tarbell, in particular, as examples of artists whose work reinforced the ideology of separate spheres.

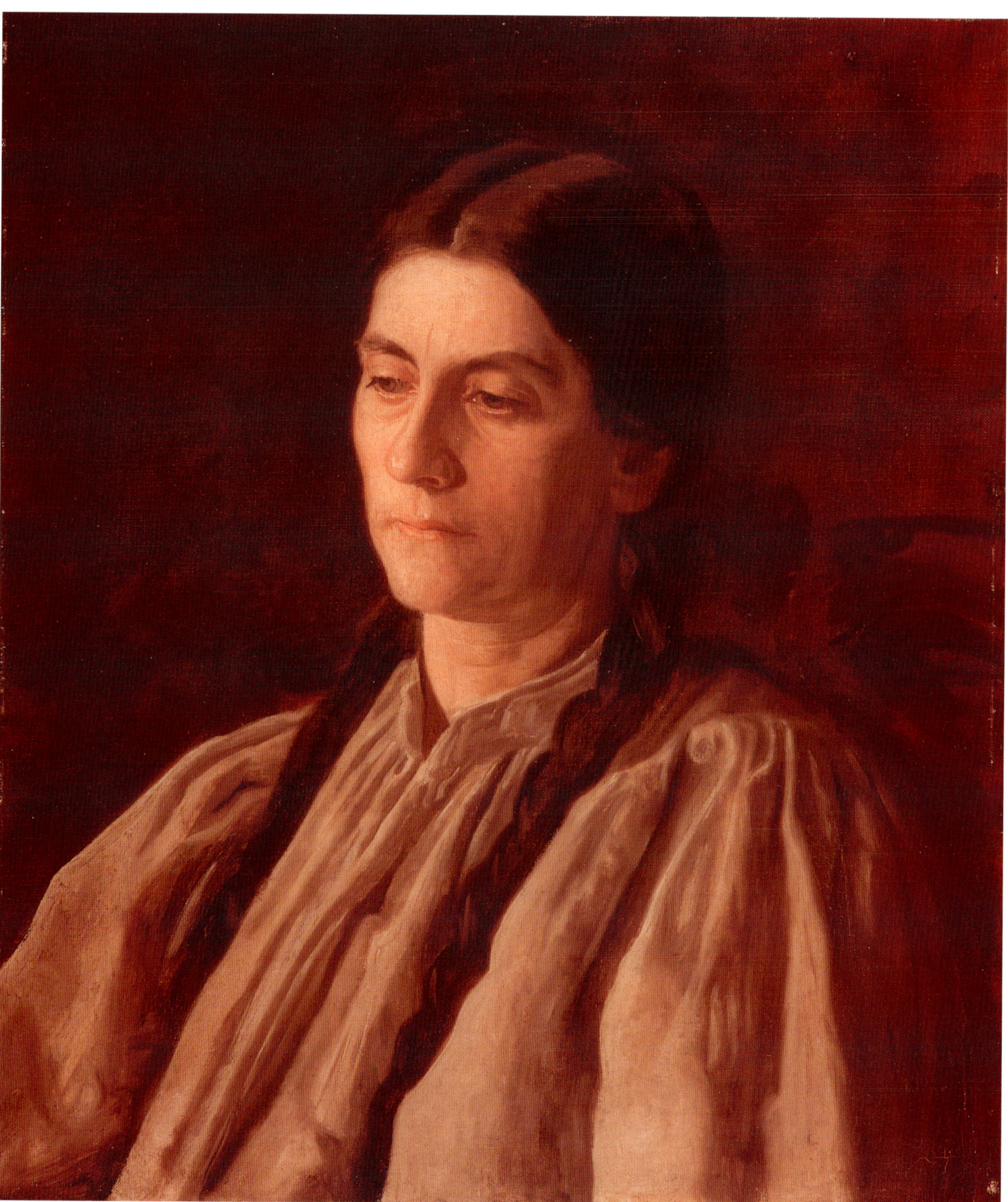

CLAIRE PERRY

AMERICAN WOMEN, NEURASTHENIA, AND THE ART OF DOING NOTHING

In 1903, the Philadelphia artist Thomas Eakins painted a portrait of Annie Williams Gandy, a close friend of the artist and his wife (fig. 40). As he had done with many other female portraits in the preceding two decades, Eakins focused on the facial expression of his sitter. He reduced the background of the painting to a blank, dark backdrop, confining the gaze of the viewer to the plain features of the woman he knew as "Mother." Eakins chose to depict Mrs. Gandy in a private moment; she is dressed in a morning coat, a robe worn at home on arising, before the rituals of dressing and the toilette were complete. The subject's long braids suggest the restfulness of the bedchamber as well as a lingering memory of her girlhood. Mrs. Gandy's weary expression and the gray, shroudlike aspect of her gown cancel out these cheering elements, however. While the painting gives us intimate access to the sitter, showing her before she has assembled the costume and coiffure of her public persona, her downcast eyes preclude any further revelations. Her firmly closed lips confirm there will be no polite conversation, offerings of tea, or other acknowledgments of the genteel rituals that governed social encounters at the turn of the century. We are allowed to view her, but "Mother" is preoccupied with interior concerns.

During the preceding two decades Eakins produced a series of paintings of female sitters in a similar vein, pictures that showed solitary women in a state of deep introspection.[1] Other artists of the period also took up the subject of the woman lost in thought, including Edmund Tarbell, a lawyer and classicist who became one of the leading painters in Boston at the time. Tarbell specialized in paintings of elegantly dressed women in sumptuous domestic settings. Unlike Eakins, who lavished attention on his female sitters' fine wrinkles and incipient jowls, Tarbell flattered his subjects with diffuse lighting and loose brushwork and by surrounding them with the opulent upholstered furnishings and bric-a-brac typical of the Gilded Age interior. Tarbell's technique erased the details of faces and bodies, calling attention instead to the overall unity of the figures, colors, and play of light in his compositions.

Around 1899, Tarbell painted *Across the Room*, a work that represented a scene of domestic repose (fig. 41). At the center of the image, a young woman sits in a ruffled

FIG. 40 [*facing*] Thomas Eakins, *Mother (Annie Williams Gandy)*, c. 1903. Oil on canvas, 24 × 20 in. Smithsonian American Art Museum. Bequest of Mrs. Lucy G. Rodman through her sister Miss Helen W. Gandy.

evening gown, the kind of dress that ladies of the leisure class wore to the fashionable dinners and balls that were part of their circuit of polite activities. She is draped across an elegant divan, slouching in a way that conveys both weariness and a disregard for the protocols of etiquette and posture her party frock implies.[2] Accentuating the sense of her distance from the world outside, the broad expanse of polished floor with the dappled texture of moving water separates the young woman from the viewer. The moatlike effect of the floor's glistening surface is complemented by the blinds on the window at the right of the canvas, which allow only diminished and fragmented sunlight to enter the room. Though the sitter's youth and formal attire mark the season of her life as one of initiation into the rituals of courtship and marriage, the isolation and lack of energy of her form, accentuated by the melancholy appearance of the cast-off garments beside her, suggest a state of mind at odds with her social circumstances. In particular, the awkward propping of the young lady's neck against the straight back of the settee speaks of a dissonance between her psychological state and the genteel entertainments her costume and surroundings represent.

Tarbell's *Across the Room* and Eakins's portrait of Mrs. Gandy were part of a larger body of paintings, prints, and photographs focusing on idle, introspective female subjects that emerged in the final decades of the nineteenth century. These representations coincided with the widespread preoccupation with the mental illness known as neurasthenia that became a national obsession during the same period. Beginning around the time of the Civil War, Americans came to believe the new habits and routines that accompanied modern industrial society were detrimental to mental and physical health. In 1860, the editors of the polite ladies' journal *Godey's Ladies' Book* warned readers that the stress and "excitement of life" in the American metropolis could lead to insanity and a "softening of the brain."[3] *A Treatise on Hygiene and Public Health*, a two-volume compendium published in 1879 that was the authoritative text on American health, also included an extended discussion on the oppressive mental influence of industrialization. In 1881, the physician George M. Beard published *American Nervousness: Its Causes and Conse-*

quences, the most widely read and influential text dealing with the link between modern life and the nervous disorder he called "neurasthenia." By the last decades of the century, neurasthenia came to be viewed as the American Disease, the illness that represented the terrible price exacted by the efficiencies and conveniences of the modern American way of life.[4]

Beard and other medical authorities believed the etiology and characteristic signs of neurasthenia were as diverse and complex as the industrial systems that provoked them. They implicated many factors in the new malady, blaming clocks, watches, the telegraph, railway travel, machine noise, and the "brain work" of office tasks and advanced study for strain on the nervous system. The physical symptoms they associated with the disease were varied, including tenderness in the scalp and gums, timidity, dyspepsia, insomnia, depression, chills, sweaty hands, dry skin, and yawning. The most typical manifestation of neurasthenia was a devastating mental and physical exhaustion that left sufferers suspended in a kind of fugue state.[5] Beard used an algebraic formula to describe the cause-and-effect relationship in the neurasthenic condition:

> Civilization in general + American civilization in particular (young and rapidly growing nation with civil, religious and social liberty) + exhausting climate (extremes of heat and cold, and dryness) + the nervous diathesis (itself a result of previously named factors) + overwork or overworry, or excessive indulgence of appetites or passions = an attack of neurasthenia or nervous exhaustion.[6]

By the 1880s, Beard and other physicians who specialized in nervous disorders claimed the sickness had reached epidemic proportions in the United States.[7] During this period the prominence and notoriety of neurasthenia inspired hundreds of articles in medical journals, as well as an avalanche of proposed remedies in advice books, newspapers, and popular journals. These sources alerted audiences to the mental scourge that was

FIG. 41 [*facing*] Edmund Charles Tarbell, *Across the Room*, c. 1899. Oil on canvas, 25 × 30⅛ in. The Metropolitan Museum of Art, Bequest of Miss Adelaide Milton de Groot (1876–1967), 1967 (67.187.141).

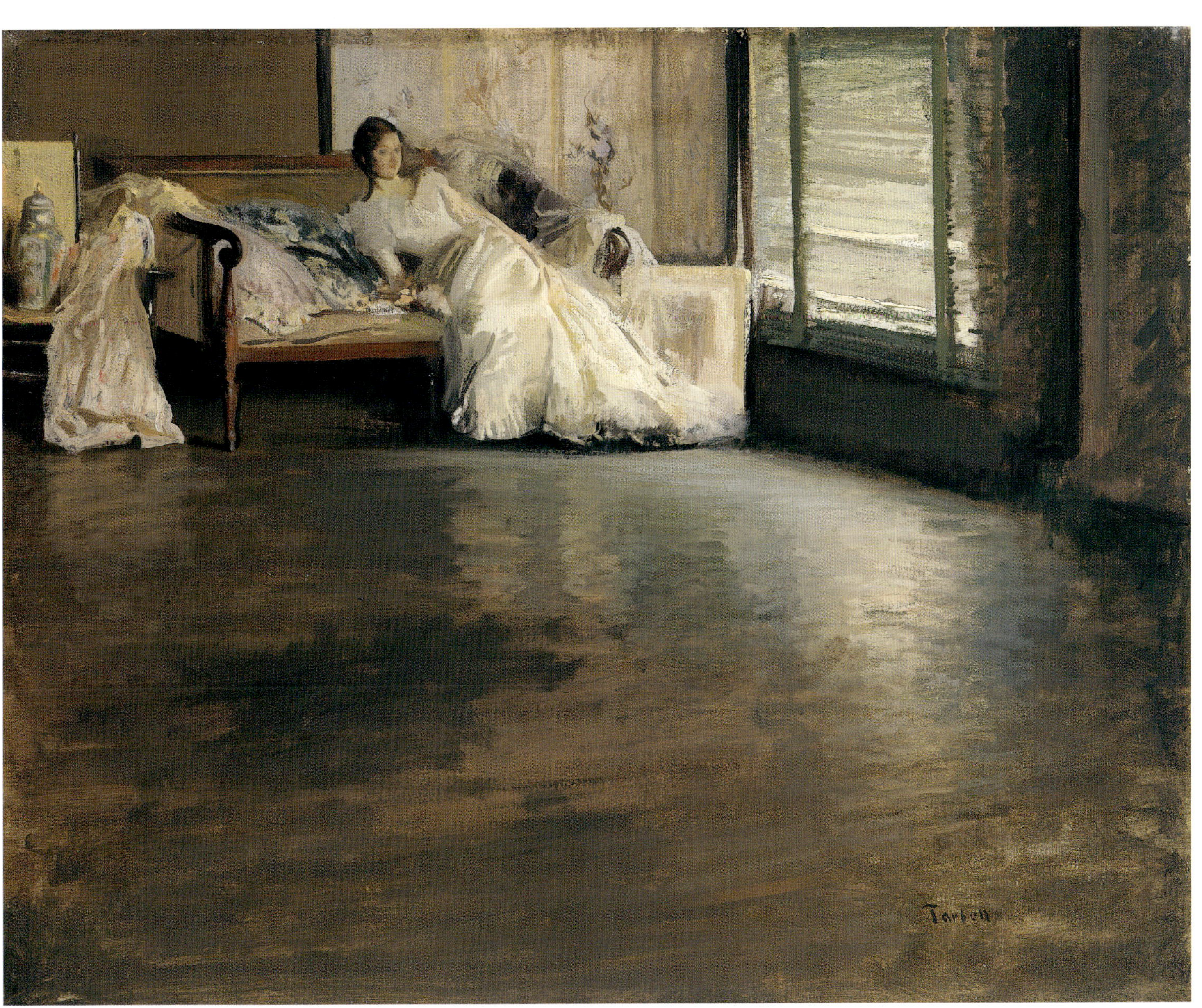

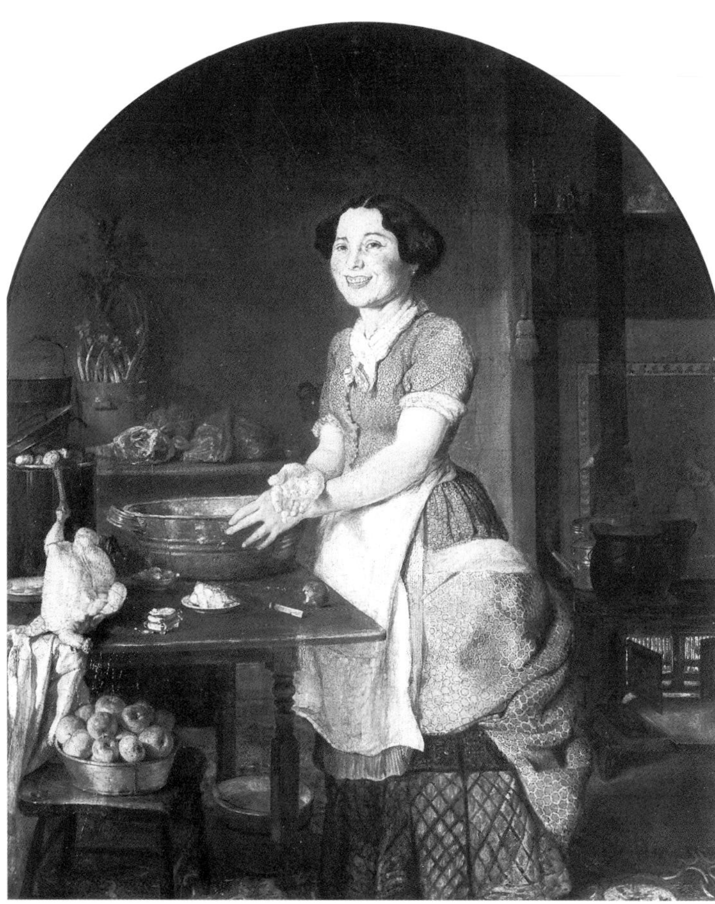

FIG. 42 Lilly Martin Spencer, *Shake Hands*, 1854. Oil on canvas, 30⅛ × 25⅛ in. Columbus: Ohio Historical Society.

sapping the strength of the nation while also helping to establish a marketing network that revolved around the disease. Advertisements with images of the afflicted invited readers to consider a profusion of treatments and therapeutic products, from hydrotherapy devices, electric stimulators, and special tonics to "rest cures" at seaside resorts offering a complete respite from urban life. Complementing this material, a collection of novels, poetry, short stories, and other literature relating to neurasthenia—written by well-known authors like Charlotte Perkins Gilman, Frank Norris, and Henry James—helped to saturate the American consciousness with the idea of the ubiquity of the disease. One writer described her own struggle with the torments of the illness:

It is the most real of all suffering. The pain of an ulcerated tooth, of a ruptured ankle ligament, of fractured ribs slips from the memory, but the anguish of the neurasthenic

state, while it becomes dulled with the passage of time, never totally disappears.... The utter lassitude of body, the weariness of the mind, the painful cerebration, the feeling as though one had committed some direful deed over night, the sense of physiologic sin, the loss of self-confidence, the depression, the accentuation of every nerve pain from which one ever suffered, in fact the utter discord and lack of harmony between the mind and the body, between oneself and the external world is well-nigh maddening.[8]

Paintings of women manifesting the physical signs of neurasthenia were an integral component of the culture that evolved around the malady during the last decades of the century. Representing the genteel aspect of American Nervousness, these works politely avoided explicit reference to the disease, though the sad eyes, delicate features, slouched posture, and general lassitude of the subjects would have been immediately recognizable to audiences as markers of neurasthenia. Portrayals of elegant sufferers helped to imbue the illness with the cachet of the social elite, as well as to define it as an affliction of women. Neurasthenia could also affect men, but women were thought to be far more susceptible because the metabolic demands of their intricate reproductive systems made the "brain work" of modern life more taxing. Medical authorities also maintained that women's access to higher education and their growing responsibilities in the public sphere, when added to the array of domestic duties, represented an untenable burden that increased the likelihood of nervous illness. A jeremiad published in a medical journal in 1889 warned American women they were "on the brink of destruction" and claimed their intellectual pursuits were incompatible with good health. "Women beware!" the author admonished his female readers. "Now you are exerting your understanding to learn Greek and solve propositions in Euclid. Beware! Oh beware!! Science pronounces that the woman who studies is lost."[9]

The neurasthenic female type in portrayals of the Gilded Age represented a radical departure from images of women created earlier in the century. When considered as part of the continuum of portrayals of American women since the Revolution, the "nervous" women in these paintings are remarkable precisely because they do nothing. Before the Civil War, American women were depicted in paintings and other imagery as the industrious helpmates of male citizens—mothers, sisters, and daughters enthusiastically engaged in shaping the nation's moral and material destiny through their devotion to domestic tasks (figs. 42 and 43). While men were represented plunging into the business of politics, investing, and taming the frontier, women were shown energetically occupied in the separate sphere of home life—caring for young children and elders, cooking, and going to market. Even formal portraits of seated women included references to their industriousness, such as floral bouquets that symbolized the number of children in the family and windows opening to views of neat farm buildings and kitchen gardens.[10] Implicit in such images was the array of virtues that American women and their work were thought to represent, such as patience, piety, filial devotion, temperance, and wisdom. Earlier in the century political leaders, authors, and clergymen had described these virtues as the natural balance to male ambition and self-interest and the moral foundation that supported the nation's democratic institutions.[11]

Like their predecessors in earlier paintings and prints, neurasthenic women functioned as the counterpart to enterprising male energies. However, rather than modeling the special virtues of the female portion of the body politic, these subjects were testaments to the physical fragility among females and the idleness that resulted from their constitutional weakness. Artists pictured the new category of American female as a delicate specimen who sat and gazed into space with an expression that communicated dreaminess, boredom, and melancholy. Conspicuously absent from such images were the domestic accoutrements emblematic of the feminine sphere in earlier paintings, including cradles, cooking pots, brooms—and well-tended husbands. In fact, the family itself is entirely absent from depictions of women curiously isolated within the empty domestic environment. A refutation of traditional female roles, the inward focus and sedentary nature of these female subjects was also an arresting counterpoint to the forward-looking ethos of an American citizenry that defined itself as a "locomotive people."[12]

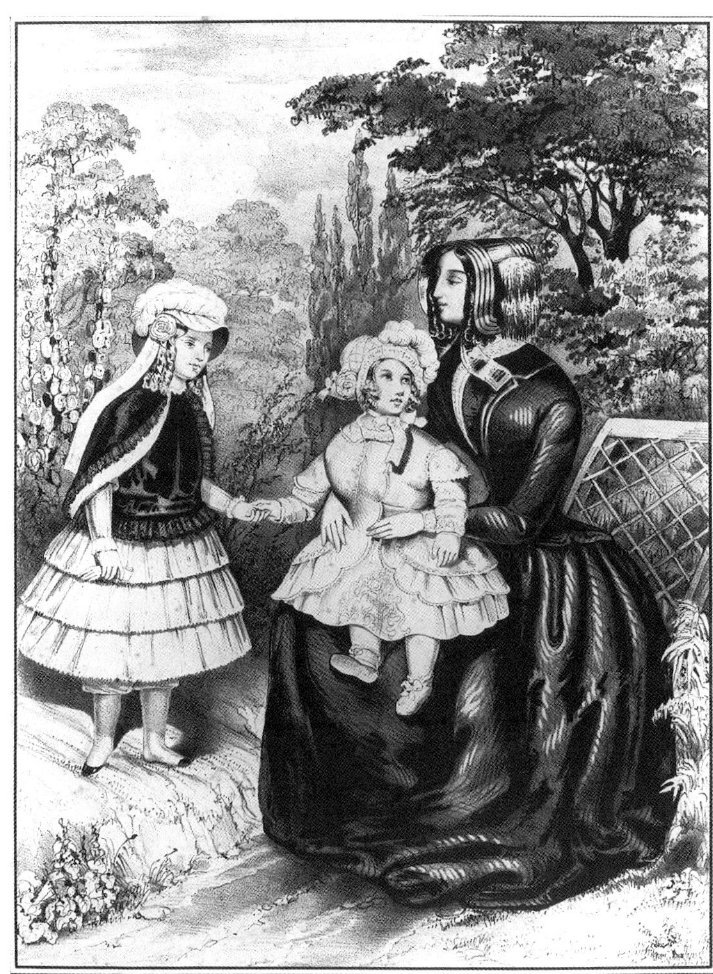

FIG. 43 Currier and Ives, Publisher, *Maternal Happiness*, 1849. Museum of the City of New York, The Harry T. Peters Collection.

The passivity of the neurasthenic type denied women's intense involvement with education, social reform, and government in the United States at the end of the nineteenth century. The period was recognized by contemporary political and religious leaders, writers, and educators as "the Era of Woman," a tribute to women's prominent role in the nation's evolving social and economic agenda. During these years women created an impressive variety of benevolent and political organizations and, through their unrelenting efforts, also succeeded in convincing the nation's colleges and universities to open their doors to female students. As part of women's new visibility in the public sphere, the question of female suffrage and the broader issue of female rights became dominant in public discourse.

Citizens engaged in heated debates about women's fitness for what the eminent Protestant minister Horace Bushnell called the "rough-hewing" work of voting and politics, activities that had remained exclusively male concerns for most of the nineteenth century.[13] Since the possibility of female political enfranchisement also pointed the way to increasing career opportunities for women as lawyers, scientists, and entrepreneurs, the subject of women's right to vote represented an array of potentially disruptive changes in the gender hierarchy that had governed American society since the Revolution.

Against the backdrop of women's shifting status, images of nervous, idle women can be understood as an expression not only of male anxieties about changes in gender relationships but also of women's awareness of the terrible impasse at which they found themselves at the end of the nineteenth century. New economic and social opportunities for women always stopped short of the ultimate confirmation of female equality and worth: the right to vote. In the context of the struggle for women's suffrage, pictures of neurasthenic types embodied the collision between women's changing perception of themselves and the prevalent belief in their inherent inferiority. Pictures of women doing "nothing" represented a moment when, in ever growing numbers, women were questioning the "cheerful obedience" of their hardworking mothers and grandmothers.[14]

Significantly, the appearance of the inactive neurasthenic woman in art coincided with a period of profound labor unrest in the United States, when the strike emerged as the favored tactic of workers protesting against their employers (fig. 44). By staging thousands of walkouts during the last quarter of the century, laborers forced many businesses to make significant concessions to their demands for higher pay and shorter workdays. Following the Great Strikes of 1877, when railroad employees crippled transportation networks across the country through a series of strikes, work stoppages became constant and highly publicized events in American life. In 1886, a year known as the "Great Upheaval," there were 1,411 significant strikes involving 9,861 companies, and roughly half of the affected companies acquiesced to the demands of strikers.[15]

Women made important contributions to late-century labor protests, in many cases through coordinated efforts between reform-minded upper- and middle-class women and female laborers. Working with organizations like the Ladies' Federal Labor Union and Knights of Labor, women who did not work for wages formed alliances with working-class women to promote a ten-hour workday, unionization, and more stringent child labor laws. The efforts of the Women's Trade Union League represented one of the most successful partnerships between working-class and well-to-do women. Women of different backgrounds came together under the auspices of the league to address problems of common concern, including women's lack of career opportunities and legal restrictions that affected women's political and economic rights. Participants in the league learned to exchange support for different causes and, through the WTUL, working-class women were enlisted to support female suffrage, a dominant issue for many middle- and upper-class members. In turn, during a massive strike of female garment workers in 1909, the league's "ladies" helped to coordinate protest shifts, joined picket lines, and were jailed along with their working-class counterparts.[16] In 1893, the Chicago socialite and reformer Bertha Honore Potter Palmer affirmed the solidarity of well-to-do women and their less fortunate sisters in an address delivered at the opening of the Women's Building at the World's Columbian Exposition: "If we can find, after a careful search, any women mounted on pedestals," she declared, "we should willingly ask them to step down— in order that they may help to uplift their sisters."[17]

Late nineteenth-century women who banded together to work for labor reforms drew on a long tradition of involvement in labor disputes that included organizing work slowdowns and stoppages. One of the earliest all-female strikes was a "turn-out" by 800 of the celebrated "mill girls" at the Lowell factory in 1834. The female operatives at the Lowell mills were renowned for their education and respectable family backgrounds, and they asserted their pedigree by linking their protests to the revered history of the American Revolution. Their petition for higher wages concluded with a poem that identified their strike with

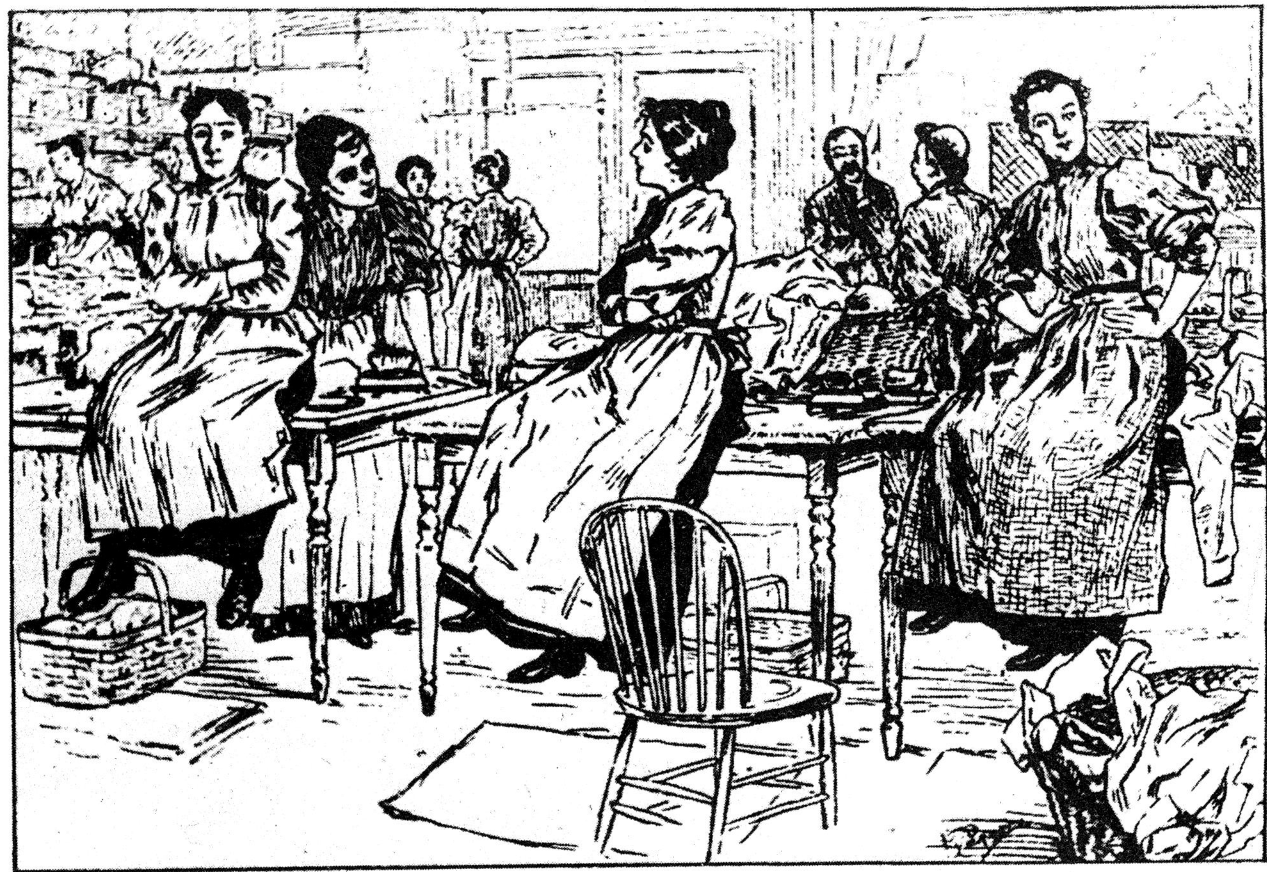

FIG. 44 *Women Workers on a Sit-Down Strike*, 1896. Pen and ink drawing. Bettman Archive.

the colonists' battle against British domination: "Yet I value not the feeble threats/of Tories in disguise," the mill workers proclaimed, "While the flag of Independence/O'er our noble nation flies."[18]

Over the next several decades, both female factory laborers and women working at home as "piece-work" seamstresses for local companies regularly used work stoppages as a means to influence their employers. The sporadic strikes of the 1830s became coordinated and ongoing efforts by mid-century, when women played a leading role in many labor protests. In 1860, 1000 female shoebinders in Lynn, Massachusetts, struck for better pay, carrying banners though the streets that proclaimed "American Ladies Will Not Be Slaves." During the Gilded Age, as the permeable economic strata of American society hardened to a significant degree, women who worked for wages—and went on strike—were typically members of the lower classes. However, the tradition of

female resistance against authority by stopping work, as well as American women's broader sense of solidarity as daughters of the Revolution, remained one of the legacies shared by all women of all classes. The relationship between striking mill girls of the 1830s, the Great Strikes of the Gilded Age, and the upper-crust ladies who malingered in fine paintings produced for elite patrons is tangled and often contradictory. However, it is clear that many American women of the Gilded Age had paused to consider their options, by looking both back to the traditions of the past and ahead toward opportunities their predecessors had helped to claim.[19]

As women at the turn of the century grappled with conflicting responsibilities and aspirations, visual representations played a pivotal role in outlining the boundaries of an emerging female identity. On one end of the spectrum were the refined neurasthenes whose frayed nerves required the cessation of female activity; at the

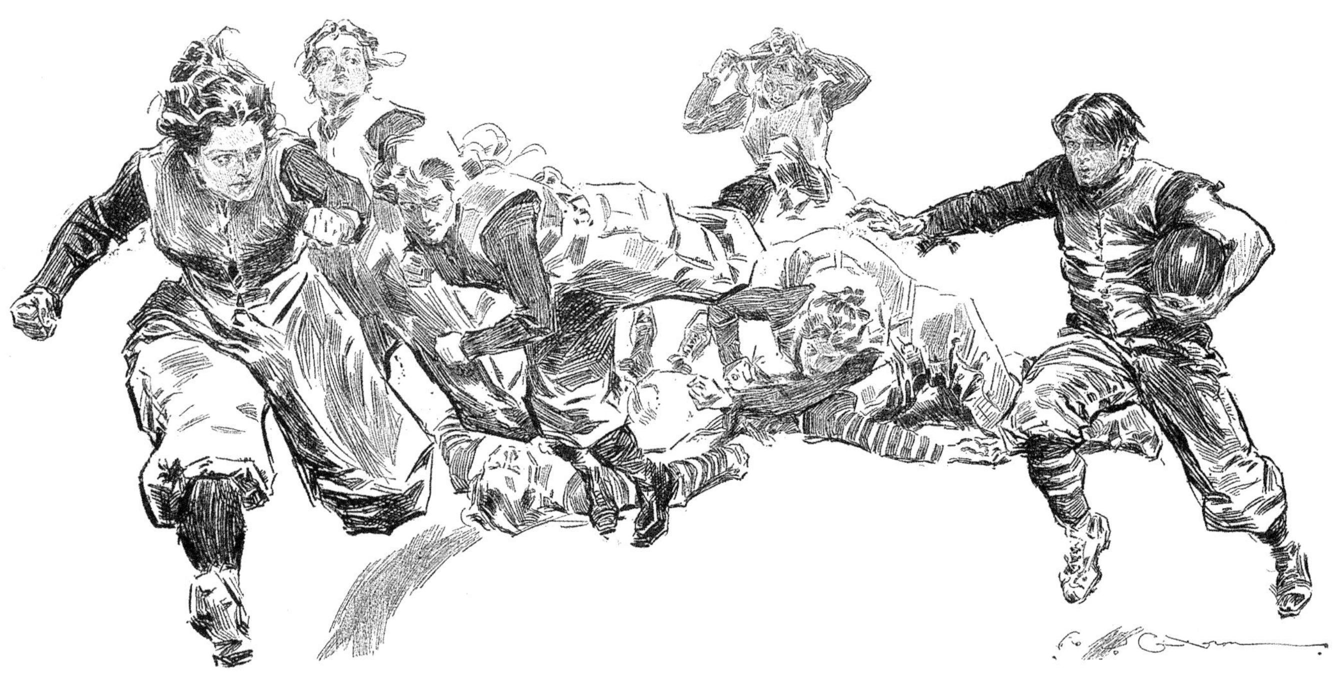

FIG. 45 Charles Dana Gibson, *The Coming Conflict*, 1896. Reprinted from
Charles Dana Gibson, *Pictures of People* (New York: Russell, 1896).

other were pictures of powerful females engaged in
political and athletic endeavors. By the 1890s, pictures
of women at suffrage rallies were a regular feature in
newspapers, and popular magazines were filled with
portrayals of the fashionably sporty, full-bodied "All-
American Girl." Made bold by the unprecedented
changes in women's sphere of activities, artists plumbed
their imaginations for creative and sometimes out-
landish visions of the new female to present to the
American public. Charles Dana Gibson, creator of the
popular "Gibson Girl," brought the genre of the empow-
ered female to its culmination—or nadir—with a
drawing titled *The Coming Conflict* (fig. 45). Executed in
1896, the image portrayed a group of determined young
women competing against male adversaries in a rousing
game of football. The ominous title of the image hinted
there were not enough rights for everyone in America,
encouraging viewers to speculate about the ultimate
meaning of female empowerment. In the new century,
it seemed, women and men would have to vie for yard-
age—jobs, political leadership, economic power—in a
zero-sum game.

Between masculinized female football players and
nervous ladies lay the contested territory where the terms
of womanhood were renegotiated at the turn of the century. The criticism inherent in both types of representations revealed the stakes of the enterprise as well as the
kinds of penalties that faced women who were exploring
new options. At the same time, the deep rift between the
two types of femininity can be understood as a symptom
of a new kind of nervousness: the dis-ease of American
men—artists, publishers, authors, physicians, clergymen, educators, and others—as they confronted female
citizens on the verge of redefining themselves.

Notes

1. For more on the subject of Eakins's late portraits, see David
M. Lubin, *Act of Portrayal: Eakins, Sargent, James* (New Haven: Yale
University Press, 1985), for his treatment of the psychological self
in Eakins's works.

2. During the nineteenth century, middle- and upper-class
Americans were keenly attuned to "good" or upright posture and
associated it with high moral standards and respectability. In this
context, the slouched posture of women depicted in many Gilded

Age portrayals embodies a disconnection from polite social conventions. For a discussion of the social significance of posture in nineteenth-century America, see the chapter "Posture and Power" in Kenneth L. Ames, *Death in the Dining Room and Other Tales of Victorian Culture* (Philadelphia: Temple University Press, 1992), 185–215; and David Yosifon and Peter N. Stearns, "The Rise and Fall of American Posture," *American Historical Review* 103, no. 4 (October 1998): 1057–95.

3. Both nineteenth-century and current literature dealing with the subject of American women's declining health during the nineteenth century is extensive. See, for example, Catherine Beecher's discussion of female health in *Treatise on Domestic Economy* (Boston: Marsh, Capen, Lyon, and Webb, 1841), 18–25; Augustus Kinsley Gardner, "The Physical Decline of American Women," *The Knickerbocker* 55, no. 1 (January 1860): 37–52; "Health in Body and Mind" in Harvey Green, *Light of the Home: An Intimate View of the Lives of Victorian Women* (New York: Pantheon Books, 1984), 131–43; and Diane Price Herndl, *Invalid Women: Figuring Female Illness in American Fiction and Culture, 1840–1940* (Chapel Hill: University of North Carolina Press, 1993).

4. In 1894, the popular journal *McClure's Magazine* defined neurasthenia as a characteristically American disease in the article "Nervousness: The National Disease of America" (February 1894): 302–7.

5. Numerous scholars have dealt with the history of neurasthenia in the United States, including Tom Lutz, *American Nervousness, 1903: An Anecdotal History* (Ithaca, NY: Cornell University Press, 1991); Nancy Tomes, *Madness in America: Cultural and Medical Perceptions of Mental Illness Before 1914* (Ithaca, NY: Cornell University Press, 1995); and Ann Douglas, "'The Fashionable Disease': Women's Complaints and Their Treatment in Nineteenth-Century America," *Journal of Interdisciplinary History* 4 (1973): 25–52.

6. George M. Beard, *American Nervousness: Its Causes and Consequences* (New York: G. P. Putnam's Sons, 1881), 176.

7. On nineteenth-century medical authorities' view that neurasthenia was pervasive in American society, see "The Price of Progress" in Francis G. Gosling, *Before Freud: Neurasthenia and the American Medical Community, 1870–1910* (Urbana: University of Illinois Press, 1987), 9–29.

8. Margaret Cleaves, MD, *The Autobiography of a Neurasthene* (Boston: The Gorham Press, 1910), 18–19.

9. Quoted in John S. Haller, Jr., "Neurasthenia: The Medical Profession and the New Woman of the Late Nineteenth Century," *New York State Journal of Medicine* (February 15, 1971): 479.

10. Dennis K. Anderson, *American Flower Painting* (New York: Watson-Guptill Publications, 1980), 10. During and after the colonial period, women were often portrayed holding sprigs of roses indicating the number of children they had borne. For more on portrayals of American women and the symbolism of flowers, see "Floral Femininity: A Pictorial Definition," *American Art* 6, no.

2 (Spring 1992): 61–78; and Judith Walsh, "The Language of Flowers in Nineteenth-Century American Painting," *The Magazine Antiques* (October 1999): 518–27.

11. Elizabeth Johns discusses nineteenth-century American art and the ideology of female virtue and separate spheres in *American Genre Painting: The Politics of Everyday Life* (New Haven: Yale University Press, 1991), 140–42.

12. Alexis de Tocqueville was one of many nineteenth-century authors who wrote about the industriousness of the American people and their orientation toward the future. See *Democracy in America* (1835; rpt. New York: Bantam Classic Book, 2000), 661–65.

13. In *The Age of Homespun: Objects and Stories in the Creation of an American Myth* (New York: Alfred A. Knopf, 2001), 12–25, Laura Thatcher Ulrich discusses Bushnell's ideas about women and politics in the United States and the broader theme of women's role in nineteenth-century America.

14. Many nineteenth-century advice books for women addressed the subject of cheerful obedience, which was promoted as one of the most important attributes of a good wife. See, for example, the chapters "Obedience" and "Cheerfulness" in William A. Alcott, *The Young Wife; or Duties of Women in the Marriage Relation* (1837; rpt., New York: Arno Press, 1972).

15. Page Smith, *The Rise of Industrial America: A People's History of the Post-Reconstruction Era*, vol. 6 (New York: Penguin Books, 1984), 223.

16. On alliances between middle-class and working-class women relating to labor issues, see Karen Manners Smith, "New Paths to Power, 1890–1920," in *No Small Courage: A History of Women in the United States*, ed. Nancy F. Cott (New York: Oxford University Press, 2000), 353–412; and Alan Trachtenberg, *The Incorporation of America: Culture and Society in the Gilded Age* (New York: Hill and Wang, 1982), 95–96.

17. Mary Kavanaugh Oldham Eagle, ed., *The Congress of Women: Held in the Women's Building, World's Columbian Exposition* (Chicago: Monarch Book Company, 1894), 27.

18. Quoted in Thomas Dublin, *Women at Work: The Transformation of Women and Work in Lowell, Massachusetts, 1826–1860* (New York: Columbia University Press, 1979), 93. For more information on the subject of striking women in the nineteenth century, see Dublin's chapters on "The Early Strikes: The 1830s" and "The Ten-Hour Movement."

19. My reading of Gilded Age portrayals of idle, introspective women draws upon and responds to scholars who see these images as evidence of the antifeminist stance of male artists and patrons. See, for example, Bernice Kramer Leader, "Antifeminism in the Paintings of the Boston School," *Arts Magazine* 56 (January 1982): 112–19. In addition to the antifeminism inherent in many late nineteenth-century images of women, I believe that women also influenced the ways in which they were portrayed in these works.

Abrams, Ann Uhry. "Frozen Goddess: The Image of Women in Nineteenth-Century Art." In *Woman's Being, Woman's Place: Female Identity and Vocation in American History*, edited by Mary Kelley, 93–108. Boston: G. K. Hall, 1979.

Apple, Rima D., ed. *Women, Health, and Medicine in America: A Historical Handbook*, 101–20. New York: Garland Publishing, Inc., 1990.

Banner, Lois W. *American Beauty: A Social History, Through Two Centuries, of the American Idea, Ideal, and Image of the Beautiful Woman*. New York: Alfred A. Knopf, 1983.

Banta, Martha. *Imaging American Women: Idea and Ideals in Cultural History*. New York: Columbia University Press, 1987.

Barker-Benfield, G. J. *The Horrors of the Half-Known Life: Male Attitudes Toward Women and Sexuality in Nineteenth-Century America*. New York: Harper & Row, 1976.

Bassuk, Ellen L. "The Rest Cure: Repetition or Resolution of Victorian Women's Conflicts?" In *The Female Body in Western Culture*, edited by Susan Rubin Suleiman. Cambridge, MA: Harvard University Press, 1986.

Bauer, Carol, and Lawrence Ritt. "'The Little Health of Ladies': An Anatomy of Female Invalidism in the Nineteenth Century." *Journal of the American Medical Women's Association* 36 (1981).

Beard, George M. *American Nervousness: Its Causes and Consequences*. New York: G. P. Putnam's Sons, 1881.

———. "Neurasthenia, or Nervous Exhaustion." *Boston Medical and Surgical Journal* 89 (1869): 217–21.

———. *Sexual Neurasthenia (Nervous Exhaustion): Its Hygiene, Causes, Symptoms, and Treatment*. New York: E. B. Treat, 1884.

Beecher, Catherine. *Treatise on Domestic Economy*, 18–25. Boston: Marsh, Capen, Lyon, and Webb, 1841.

Betsky, Celia. "In the Artist's Studio." *Portfolio* 4, no. 1 (January/February 1982): 32–39.

Bresnahan, Keith. "Neurasthenic Subjects and the Bourgeois Interior." *Space & Culture* 6, no. 2 (May 2003): 169–77.

Bromberg, Joan Jacobs. "Chlorotic Girls, 1870–1920: A Historical Perspective on Female Adolescence." *Child Development* 53 (1982): 1468–77.

Buckley, Laurene. *Edmund C. Tarbell: Poet of Domesticity*. New York: Hudson Hills Press, 2001.

Burns, Sarah. *Inventing the Modern Artist: Art and Culture in the Gilded Age*. New Haven: Yale University Press, 1996.

———. "The Poetic Mode in American Painting: George Fuller and Thomas Dewing." PhD diss., University of Illinois, Urbana-Champaign, 1979.

———. "Revitalizing the 'Painted Out' North: Winslow Homer, Manly Health, and New England Regionalism in Turn-of-the-Century America." *American Art* 9, no. 2 (Summer 1995).

Call, Annie Payson. *Power Through Repose*. Boston: Roberts Brothers, 1891.

Chopin, Kate. *The Awakening and Selected Stories*. 1899. Reprint, New York: Penguin Books, 1984.

Cleaves, Margaret. *The Autobiography of a Neurasthene*. Boston: The Gorham Press, 1910.

———. "Neurasthenia and Its Relation to Diseases of Women." *Transactions of the Iowa State Medical Association* 9 (1886): 166–67.

Cogan, Frances B. *All-American Girl: The Ideal of Real Womanhood in Mid-Nineteenth-Century America*. Athens: University of Georgia Press, 1989.

Cott, Nancy F., ed. *History of Women in the United States*, volume 2, 298–315. Munich: K. G. Saut, 1993.

———. *No Small Courage: A History of Women in the United States*. New York: Oxford University Press, 2000.

Courtney, J. W. "Hygiene of the Brain and Nervous System." In *A Manual of Personal Hygiene: Proper Living Upon a Physiological Basis*, edited by Walter L. Pyle, 300. Philadelphia: W. B. Saunders, 1901.

Dana, Charles L. "The Partial Passing of Neurasthenia." *Boston Medical and Surgical Journal* 150 (1904): 339–44.

Davis, Richard Harding. "Charles Dana Gibson's Pictures: The Origins of a Type of the American Girl." *Monthly Illustrator* 3 (January 3, 1895): 6.

Douglas, Ann. "'The Fashionable Disease': Women's Complaints and Their Treatment in Nineteenth-Century America." *Journal of Interdisciplinary History* 4 (1973).

Drinka, George Frederick. *The Birth of Neurosis: Myth, Malady and the Victorians*. New York: Simon & Schuster, 1984.

Dublin, Thomas. *Women at Work: The Transformation of Women and Work in Lowell, Massachusetts, 1826–1860*. New York: Columbia University Press, 1979.

Duby, Georges, and Michelle Perot. *Power and Beauty: Images of Women in Art.* London: Tauris Parke Books, 1992.

Ehrenreich, Barbara, and Deirdre English. *For Her Own Good: 150 Years of the Experts' Advice to Women.* New York: Anchor Press/Doubleday, 1978.

Fairbrother, Trevor J. *The Bostonians, Painters of an Elegant Age.* Boston: Museum of Fine Arts, 1986.

Fellman, Anita Clair, and Michael Fellman. *Making Sense of Self: Medical Advice Literature in Late Nineteenth-Century America.* Philadelphia: University of Pennsylvania Press, 1981.

Figlio, Karl. "Chlorosis and Chronic Disease in Nineteenth-Century Britain: The Social Constitution of Somatic Illness in a Capitalist Society." *Social History* 3 (May 1978): 167–97.

Fryer, Judith. "Women and Space: The Flowering of Desire." *Prospects* 9 (1984): 187–230.

Gammel, R. H. Ives. *The Boston Painters, 1900–1930.* Orleans, MA: Parnassus Imprints, 1986.

Gardner, Augustus Kinsley. "Health in Body and Mind." In *Light of the Home: An Intimate View of the Lives of Victorian Women,* edited by Harvey Green. New York: Pantheon Books, 1984.

———. "The Physical Decline of American Women." *The Knickerbocker* 55, no. 1 (January 1860).

Gibson, Charles Dana. *The Gibson Book: A Collection of the Published Works of Charles Dana Gibson.* New York: Scribner's Sons, 1906.

Gilman, Charlotte Perkins. *The Yellow Wallpaper.* 1892. Reprint, Old Westbury, NY: The Feminist Press, 1973.

———. "Why I Wrote the Yellow Wallpaper." *The Forerunner* 4 (October 1913).

Goodrich, Lloyd. *Thomas Eakins.* Washington, D.C.: The National Gallery of Art, 1982.

Gordon, Beverly. "Woman's Domestic Body: The Conceptual Conflation of Women and Interiors in the Industrial Age." *Winterthur Portfolio* 30, no. 1 (Spring 1995): 281–99.

Gosling, Francis G. *Before Freud: Neurasthenia and the American Medical Community, 1870–1910.* Urbana: University of Illinois Press, 1987.

Haller, John S., Jr. "Neurasthenia: The Medical Profession and the New Woman of the Late Nineteenth Century." *New York State Journal of Medicine* (February 15, 1971): 479.

Haller, Robin M., and John S. Haller, Jr. *The Physician and Sexuality in Nineteenth-Century America.* Urbana: University of Illinois Press, 1974.

Hartman, Mary S., and Lois Banner. *Clio's Consciousness Raised: New Perspectives on the History of Women.* New York: Harper Collins Books, 1974.

Hendricks, Gordon. *The Life and Work of Thomas Eakins.* New York: Grossman Publishers, 1974.

Herndl, Diane Price. *Invalid Women: Figuring Female Illness in American Fiction and Culture, 1840–1940.* Chapel Hill: University of North Carolina Press, 1993.

Hirshler, Erica E. "Lillian W. Hale: Women and the Boston School." PhD diss., Boston University, 1990.

Hobbs, Susan A. *The Art of Thomas Wilmer Dewing: Beauty Reconfigured.* Washington, D.C.: The Smithsonian Institution Press, in association with The Brooklyn Museum, 1996.

Hoeksema, Susan Nolan. "Epidemiology and Theories of Gender Differences in Unipolar Depression." In *Gender and Psychopathology,* edited by Mary V. Seeman, Washington, D.C.: American Psychiatric Press, Inc., 1995.

Hoppin, Augustus. *A Fashionable Sufferer; or, Chapters from Life's Comedy.* New York: Houghton, Mifflin and Company, 1883.

Hunter, Jane H. *How Young Ladies Became Girls: The Victorian Origins of American Girlhood.* New Haven: Yale University Press, 2002.

Hunter, Richard, and Ida Macalpine. *Three Hundred Years of Psychiatry.* 1963. Reprint, London: Oxford University Press, 1970.

Jennings, Gertrude E. "A Rest Cure." In *Four One-Act Plays,* 11–34. New York: Samuel French, 1914.

Jewell, James S. "The Varieties and Causes of Neurasthenia." *The Journal of Nervous and Mental Disease* 7 (1880): 1–16.

Kessler, Ronald. "Gender Differences in the Prevalence and Correlates of Mood Disorders in the General Population." In *Mood Disorders in Women,* edited by Meir Steiner, Kimberly Yonkers, and Elias Eriksson. London: Martin Dunitz, 2000.

Kimmel, Michael. "Men's Responses to Feminism at the Turn of the Century." *Gender and Society* 1 (September 1987): 261–83.

Kitch, Carolyn. *The Girl on the Magazine Cover: The Origins of Visual Stereotypes in American Mass Media.* Chapel Hill: University of North Carolina Press, 2001.

Koch, Robert. "Gibson Girl Revisited." *Art in America* 53 (1965).

Leader, Bernice Kramer. "Antifeminism in the Paintings of the Boston School." *Arts Magazine* 56 (January 1982): 112–19.

———. "The Boston Lady as a Work of Art: Paintings by the Boston School at the Turn of the Century." PhD diss., Columbia University, 1980.

Lears, T. J. Jackson. *No Place of Grace: Antimodernism and the Transformation of American Culture, 1880–1920.* New York: Pantheon Books, 1981.

Lee, Ellen Wardwell. *William McGregor Paxton.* Indianapolis: Indianapolis Museum of Art, 1979.

Lifton, Norma. "Thomas Eakins and S. Weir Mitchell: Images in Cures in the Late Nineteenth Century." *Psychoanalytic Perspectives on Art* 2 (1987): 247–74.

Longshore-Potts, Mrs. A. M. *Discourses to Women on Medical Subjects.* San Diego: Published by the author, 1896.

Lubin, David M. *Act of Portrayal: Eakins, Sargent, James.* New Haven: Yale University Press, 1985.

———. "Modern Psychological Selfhood in the Art of Thomas Eakins." In *Inventing the Psychological: Toward a Cultural History of Emotional Life in America,* edited by Joel Pfister and Nancy Schnog, 133–66. New Haven: Yale University Press, 1997.

Lutz, Tom. *American Nervousness, 1903: An Anecdotal History.* Ithaca, NY: Cornell University Press, 1991.

Lyczko, Judith Elizabeth. "Thomas Wilmer Dewing's Sources: Women in Interiors." *Arts Magazine* 54, no. 3 (September 1979).

Maxwell, William B. *The Rest Cure, a Novel.* New York: Appleton, 1910.

McReynolds, Rosalee. "The Sexual Politics of Illness in Turn-of-the-Century Libraries." *Libraries and Culture* 25 (Spring 1990): 194–217.

Merikangas, Kathleen. "Epidemiology of Mood Disorders in Women." In *Mood Disorders in Women*, edited by Mein Steiner, Kimberly Yonkers, and Elias Eriksson, 1–14. London: Martin Dunitz, 2000.

Meyer, Donald. *The Positive Thinkers: Popular Religious Psychology from Mary Baker Eddy to Norman Vincent Peale and Ronald Reagan.* Middletown, CT: Wesleyan University Press, 1988.

Mitchell, S. Weir. "Clinical Lecture on Nervousness in the Male." *The Medical News and Library* 35 (December 1877).

———. *Doctor and Patient.* Philadelphia: J. B. Lippincott & Co., 1888.

———. *Fat and Blood: An Essay on the Treatment of Certain Forms of Neurasthenia and Hysteria.* London: J. B. Lippincott & Co., 1891.

———. *Wear and Tear, or Hints for the Overworked.* Philadelphia: J. B. Lippincott & Co., 1871.

Moore, Sarah J. *John White Alexander and the Construction of National Identity: Cosmopolitan American Art, 1880–1915.* Newark: University of Delaware Press, 2003.

Morgan, Jayne. "Edward Muybridge and W. S. Playfair: An Aesthetics of Neurasthenia." *History of Photography* 23 (Autumn 1999): 225–31.

Mrozek, Donald J. "The 'Amazon' and the American 'Lady': Sexual Fears of Women as Athletes." In *From Fair Sex to Feminism: Sport and the Socialization of Women in the Industrial and Post-Industrial Eras*, edited by J. A. Mangan and Roberta J. Park. London: Frank Cass and Co., 1987.

"Nervousness: The National Disease of America." *McClure's Magazine* (February 1894): 302–7.

Nochlin, Linda. "Issues of Gender in Cassatt and Eakins." In *Nineteenth-Century Art: A Critical History*, edited by Stephen F. Eisenman et al., 5–73. London: Thames and Hudson, 1994.

Parker, Gail Thain. *Mind Cure in New England: From the Civil War to World War I.* Hanover, NH: University Press of New England, 1973.

Pierce, Patricia Jobe. *Edmund C. Tarbell and the Boston School of Painting, 1889–1980.* New York: Hacker Art Books, 1980.

Pitz, Henry C. "Charles Dana Gibson: Creator of a Mode." *American Artist* 20 (December 1956): 50–55.

Porter, Roy. "The Body and the Mind, the Doctor and the Patient." In *Hysteria Beyond Freud*, edited by Sander L. Gilman, Helen King, Roy Porter, G. S. Rousseau, and Elaine Showalter. Berkeley: University of California Press, 1993.

Pyne, Kathleen. *Art and the Higher Life: Painting and Evolutionary Thought in Late Nineteenth-Century America.* Austin: University of Texas Press, 1996.

———. "Evolutionary Typology and the American Woman in the Work of Thomas Wilmer Dewing." *American Art* 7 (Fall 1993): 13–30.

Rein, David S. *S. Weir Mitchell as a Psychiatric Novelist.* New York: International Universities Press, 1952.

Robinson, Joyce Henri. "'Hi honey, I'm home': Weary (Neurasthenic) Businessmen and the Formulation of a Serenely Modern Aesthetic." In *Not at Home: The Suppression of Domesticity in Modern Art and Architecture*, edited by Christopher Reed. London: Thames & Hudson, 1996.

Rogers, Agnes. "The Undimmed Appeal of the Gibson Girl." *American Heritage* 9 (December 1957).

Rotondo, Anthony E. *American Manhood: Transformations in Masculinity from the Revolution to the Modern Era.* New York: Basic Books, 1993.

Rozinek, Erika Ingelin. "'We All Take Our Turn': Invalidism in American Culture, 1850–1910." Master's thesis, University of Delaware, 2003.

Ruddock, E. H. *The Lady's Manual of Homeopathic Treatment in the Various Derangements Incident to her Sex*, 9th edition. New York: Boericke and Tafel, 1886.

Sadler, William S. *Worry and Nervousness: The Science of Self-Mastery.* Chicago: A. C. McClurg & Co., 1914.

Showalter, Elaine. *The Female Malady: Women, Madness, and English Culture, 1830–1980.* New York: Pantheon Books, 1985.

Sicherman, Barbara. "The Paradox of Prudence: Mental Health in the Gilded Age." *The Journal of American History* 62, no. 4 (March 1976): 890–912.

———. "The Uses of a Diagnosis: Doctors, Patients, and Neurasthenia." *Journal of the History of Medicine* 32 (1977): 33–45.

Smith-Rosenberg, Carroll. "The New Woman as Androgyne: Social Disorder and Gender Crisis, 1870–1936." In *Disorderly Conduct: Visions of Gender in Victorian America*, 245–96. New York: Alfred A. Knopf, 1985.

Smith-Rosenberg, Carroll, and Charles Rosenberg. "The Female Animal: Medical and Biological Views of Woman and Her Role in Nineteenth-Century America." *Journal of American History* 60 (September 1973): 332–56.

Springer, Julie Anne. "Art and the Feminine Muse: Women in Interiors by John White Alexander." *Woman's Art Journal* 6, no. 2 (Fall 1985/Winter 1986): 1–8.

Stage, Sarah. *Female Complaints: Lydia Pinkham and the Business of Women's Medicine.* New York: W. W. Norton & Co., Inc., 1979.

Stea, John. "Remedies for Society's Debilities: Medicines for Neurasthenia in Victorian America." *New York State Journal of Medicine* 93 (1993).

Stott, Annette. "Floral Femininity: A Pictorial Definition." *American Art* 6, no. 2 (Spring 1992).

Strouse, Jean. *Alice James, a Biography*. Boston: Houghton Mifflin, 1980.

Stuart, Ruth McEnery. *The Cocoon: A Rest-Cure Comedy*. New York: Hearst's International Library Co., 1915.

Theriot, Nancy M. "Psychosomatic Illness in History: The 'Green Sickness' Among Nineteenth-Century Adolescent Girls." *The Journal of Psychohistory* 15 (Spring 1998): 461–80.

Todd, Ellen Wiley. *The "New Woman" Revised: Painting and Gender Politics on Fourteenth Street*. Berkeley: University of California Press, 1993.

Tomes, Nancy. *Madness in America: Cultural and Medical Perceptions of Mental Illness Before 1914*. Ithaca, NY: Cornell University Press, 1995.

Truettner, William. "Dressing the Part: Thomas Eakins' *Portrait of Frank Hamilton Cushing*." *American Art Journal* 17 (Spring 1985).

Van Hook, Bailey. *Angels of Art: Women and Art in American Society, 1876–1914*. University Park: The Pennsylvania State University Press, 1996.

———. "Decorative Images of American Women: The Aristocratic Aesthetic of the Late Nineteenth Century." *Smithsonian Studies in American Art* 4 (Winter 1990): 45–69.

———. "'Milk White Angels of Art': Images of Women in Turn-of-the-Century America." *Woman's Art Journal* (Fall 1990/Winter 1991): 23–29.

Veith, Ilza. *Hysteria: The History of a Disease*. Chicago: University of Chicago Press, 1965.

Weibel, Kathryn. *Mirror Mirror: Images of Women Reflected in Popular Culture*. Garden City, NY: Anchor Books, 1977.

Wilmerding, John, ed. *Thomas Eakins and the Heart of American Life*. London: The National Portrait Gallery, 1993.

Wolstenholme, Susan. "Edith Wharton's Gibson Girl: The Virgin, the Undine, and the Dynamo." *American Literary Realism* 18 (1985).

11; psychological, 11; rest cure as, 1, 2, 11, 13, 23, 50n27, 72; self-control as, 25–26, 27, 33; surgery as, 10
Ticknor, Caroline, "The Steel-Engraving Lady and the Gibson Girl," 53–54, 62
Treatise on Hygiene and Public Health, A, 70

Utamaro, Kitagawa, 22

Van Buren, Amelia, 40, 49n16
Veblen, Thorstein, 48
Vermeer, Johannes, 22, 33

weariness, chronic. *See* neurasthenia
Weir, Julian Alden, 33; *A Gentlewoman*, 28, **28**
Wharton, Edith, 38, 48
Whistler, James McNeill, influence of, 22, 30
Wiles, Irving Ramsay, 26
Willard, Frances, 10
Winchester's Specific Pill, 38

Woman at Home: antifeminism and, 33n1; as genre, 4, 22, 25, 26, 28, 30, 33, 33n1, 63; as ideology, 2, 21, 23, 73
women: changing social roles of, 1–2, 5, 10, 13, 33, 33n1, 53, 55, 63, 73–74, 75–76; control of, 50n31, 59–60; dangers of education for, 9–10, **12**, 72; eroticization of sick, 4, 43–44; images of, 54–55, 70, 72–73, 77n10; major depression and, 13; neurasthenic, as dangerous, 43–44; reproductive system of, and neurasthenia, 8–9, 38, 72; stereotyping of, 2, 4; as susceptible to neurasthenia, 1, 2, 4, 6, 8, 38, 72; withdrawn, as artistic trope, 4
Women's Christian Temperance Union, 10
Women's Trade Union League (WTUL), 74
Women Workers on a Sit-Down Strike, **75**
Wood, Dr. Horatio, 42
WTUL. *See* Women's Trade Union League

Yellow Wall-paper, The, **3**
youth, gender conflict in, 45–46

PRODUCED BY WILSTED & TAYLOR PUBLISHING SERVICES

Production management and art direction: Christine Taylor

Copy editing: Rachel Bernstein

Design and composition: Melissa Ehn

Printing and binding in Hong Kong:
Regal Printing Ltd. through Stacy Quinn
of QuinnEssentials Books and Printing, Inc.